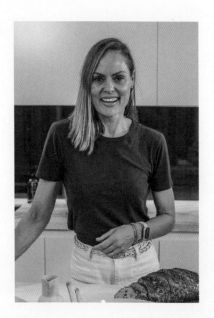

Zoe Bingley-Pullin is one of Australia's most trusted nutritionists – a chef, presenter and author with over 20 years' experience in the nutrition industry and in private practice. A recognised media personality across television, print and digital, Zoe was co-host of *Good Chef Bad Chef* (Network Ten) for five seasons and in 2017 joined *The House of Wellness* as segment host (Seven Network), which in 2018 expanded to her being a regular guest host on *The House of Wellness* TV and radio show.

Zoe has a strong vision to empower women with the knowledge and tools needed to navigate perimenopause and menopause. Working with many brands as an expert nutritionist, Zoe engages with her social media audience to promote brand messaging and is currently an ambassador and nutritional expert for Woolworths Bunch Community and an ongoing Cure Cancer Ambassador.

EAT YOUR WAY TO HEALTHY HORMONES

ZOE BINGLEY-PULLIN

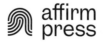

affirm press

Contents

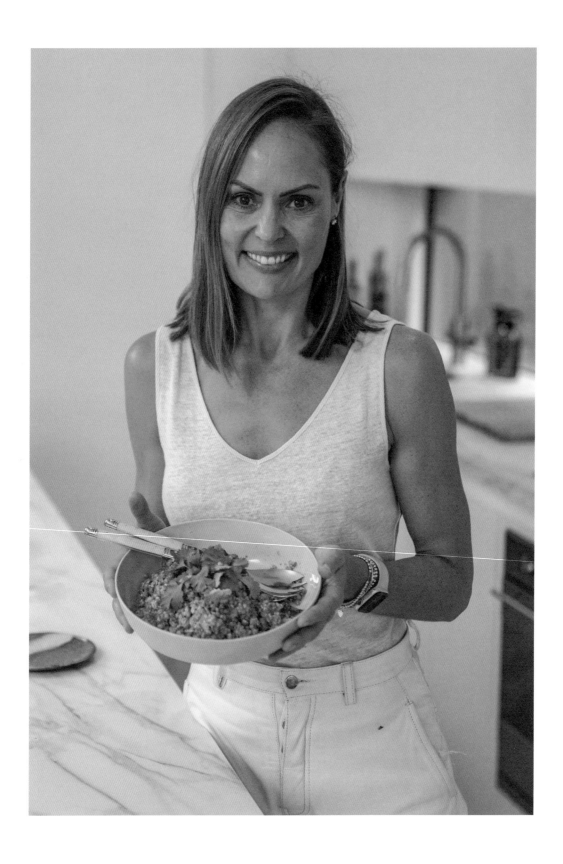

Introduction

I thought I was going 'mad' and my body had turned against me.

I never thought I would be perimenopausal at 39. I was giving IVF one last shot, after many failed attempts to have a second child.

My doctor saw my blood test results and told me I had a 2 per cent chance of falling pregnant.

There it was, all the signs were pointing toward perimenopausal.

It all made sense now: why my periods were irregular, why my breasts were sore and swollen and why I would cry at the drop of a hat.

This was a turning point for me – a not-so-gentle reminder that it was time to take control of my hormones. No longer would I allow them to be in control of me.

With over 20 years' experience as a registered and practising nutritionist in the nutrition and wellness industry, what I found so amazing was the lack of understanding and conversation around perimenopause. Where in hindsight most often the symptoms were not recognised and overlapped with other common health issues, even my own focus in practice had been more on hormones for weight loss rather than general health.

I jumped into understanding hormones headfirst and have spent the last six years devouring as much information as possible. I went back to study, I learned more about pathology results and how to clearly understand hormone blood results, I learned more about pharmacology and what medication people were taking. I read medical publications, attended seminars and webinars, talked to my clients and even did a course on psychotherapy to help teach people how to identify when they are overwhelmed and how to process those feelings, and I combined all this with my past experience from working with my clients.

I personally started having regular blood tests to look at my hormones and worked out which foods and supplements would best support me. I changed my exercise to best support my nervous system. I started meditating regularly and owning up to my anxiety and depression. I asked for more help without feeling ashamed and embarrassed and I talked and talked and talked about my body to my girlfriends and asked them questions about theirs.

As a result, I now have the knowledge, tools and drive to manage my hormonal health, which has turned things around and given me a new chapter of my life of my own design. After not having a second child and learning more about perimenopause, it has become my mission to inspire others to get comfortable with the uncomfortable and untangle the web of their own hormones.

I have written this book to support you on your journey to optimal hormonal health – and yes, it is achievable!

In the first part of the book, I explain what hormones are and how they affect us at different stages in our lives, from our tweens to old age. I haven't included children under nine because their hormones don't fluctuate as much – a balanced, healthy diet is all they need to help them grow.

In these pages, you will find my heartfelt guidance on how, what and when to eat to keep your hormones in balance at any age. I'll look at some common health issues caused by hormone imbalance and how to manage them, and share tips from experts about other strategies you can use to stay in control, such as breathing exercises, meditation and simple yoga poses.

I share some of my own experiences along the way, and I've also included case studies of clients I have successfully supported to address their hormonal issues.

This is first and foremost a recipe book, though, and the second part is dedicated to delicious, nourishing and simple-to-follow recipes. There are chapters for smoothies and juices, breakfast, lunch, dinner, sauces and sides, and sweets, all of them designed to make eating well easier and have you and your family feeling your best. Be sure to look at the recipe tips – they'll give you handy hints about everything from boosting muscle mass to managing hot flushes and much more in between.

I hope *Eat Your Way to Healthy Hormones* will give you greater insight into the relationship between hormones and diet, and why what we put into our mouths and bodies matters when it comes to hormonal health.

Hormonal Health Basics

A Primer on Hormones

We blame our hormones for everything: from stress and slow metabolism to mood swings, painful periods and even a low libido. They're why we binge on sugar and chocolate, slam doors and develop 'midlife spread'. But what exactly are hormones?

What are hormones?

Hormones are chemical messengers produced by a network of glands and organs called the endocrine system and circulated to other parts of the body via the bloodstream to regulate their function. For example, oestrogen, which has important functions in reproduction, is produced in the ovaries, and the pancreas produces insulin, which helps the body regulate blood sugars. Hormones control many of our most important physiological processes, including metabolism, growth, reproduction and mood. We often describe teenagers as 'hormonal', but hormones are present in all of us – young and old alike.

What do hormones do?

Hormones play crucial roles in various physiological processes in the body, and while many hormones have specific functions, there can be some overlap or interactions between them. Different hormones work together in a complex, coordinated manner to maintain our overall health and keep our bodies working.

Here is a basic overview of some important hormones and their functions:

Cortisol: Often referred to as the 'stress hormone', cortisol helps the body respond to stress and regulates various metabolic processes. It can influence blood pressure, immune function and the body's response to inflammation.

Follicle Stimulating Hormone (FSH): FSH is a key player in the reproductive system, helping to regulate the production of eggs in females and sperm in males. FSH is essential for the maturation of follicles in the ovaries and the development of the testes.

Ghrelin: Ghrelin is a hormone produced in the stomach that stimulates hunger and promotes food intake. Often referred to as the 'hunger hormone', ghrelin levels typically rise before meals and decrease after eating, influencing appetite and meal initiation.

Growth Hormone: This hormone, produced by the pituitary gland, stimulates growth and cell reproduction. It's especially important during childhood and adolescence for proper development.

Insulin: Insulin is a hormone produced by the pancreas that regulates blood sugar levels by facilitating the uptake of glucose into cells. It plays a crucial role in maintaining glucose homeostasis and energy metabolism.

Luteinising Hormone (LH): LH plays a pivotal role in reproduction. In females, it triggers ovulation and stimulates the production of progesterone. In males, it stimulates the testes to produce testosterone. LH, along with FSH, helps to regulate the menstrual cycle in women.

Melatonin: Melatonin, produced in the pineal gland, is the hormone responsible for regulating our sleep–wake cycle. It increases in the evening to prepare the body for sleep and decreases in the morning to help wake us up.

Oestrogen: Both women and men have oestrogen, though men have it in smaller amounts. Oestrogen plays a key role in the development of female sexual characteristics, regulating the menstrual cycle and maintaining bone health.

Progesterone: Progesterone is crucial to the female reproductive system. It helps regulate the menstrual cycle, prepares the uterus for pregnancy and supports the early stages of pregnancy.

Serotonin: Serotonin is a neurotransmitter that contributes to mood regulation, sleep and appetite. It is often referred to as the 'feel-good' neurotransmitter, and imbalances in serotonin levels have been linked to conditions such as depression and anxiety.

Testosterone: Testosterone is the primary male sex hormone; women have testosterone too, but not as much. It's responsible for male sexual development and building muscle and bone mass. It also plays a role in mood and energy levels.

What causes hormonal imbalance?

Think of your hormones as an orchestra – you want them playing together. If one is off beat, it can throw out the whole rhythm, causing us to experience unwanted symptoms.

Things that can throw your hormones out of kilter include poor diet or extreme dieting, excessive alcohol, chronic stress, too much high-intensity exercise, poor gut health, insufficient sleep ... and the list goes on and on!

Hormone imbalances can have an immense impact on our physical, mental and emotional wellbeing, with symptoms such as fatigue, depression and infertility. We are all vulnerable to hormone dysregulation, though women are more prone to it than men.

But despite its complexities, managing our hormones does not have to go into the too-hard basket. We can take control of our hormonal health. Understanding the relationship between food and hormones is a good place to start, but diet isn't the only way that we can take charge.

The five areas of focus

In 20 years working as a nutritionist, I have seen firsthand the benefits of adopting a holistic approach to hormonal health. A holistic approach is one that considers a person's mental, emotional, social and spiritual wellbeing as well as their physical wellbeing, seeing them all as intertwined.

What we eat, how we move and even how we think and feel affect our hormones. In my practice, I focus on five different areas that influence my clients' hormonal health: nutrition, movement, mind, connection and conventional medicine. In the next few chapters, we'll look at these five areas and why they're so important.

Nutrition

Eat your way to healthy hormones

Nutrition is the foundation of health at the cellular level. The body relies on a variety of nutrients, including vitamins, minerals and amino acids, to synthesise and regulate hormones, so what we eat has a profound impact on our hormonal health. A well-balanced and nutrient-dense diet that includes a variety of whole foods can help support healthy hormone production, regulation and balance, while a poor diet can contribute to hormonal imbalances and associated health issues.

These health issues can include:

Poor gut health: The gut is often referred to as the 'second brain', because it houses an extensive network of neurons and produces various hormones, including serotonin and ghrelin. Diet profoundly affects the gut microbiome and gut hormone levels, which can, in turn, influence mood, appetite and even thyroid function.

Uncontrolled blood sugar: Foods with a high glycaemic load, such as refined sugars and processed carbohydrates, have a direct impact on blood sugar levels. Uncontrolled blood sugar levels can lead to insulin resistance, a condition associated with the development of type 2 diabetes. Two common ways to measure how carbohydrate-containing foods impact our blood sugar are the glycaemic index (GI) and glycaemic load (GL):

- GI ranks carbs on how quickly they break down into sugar in the blood: a high GI (70+) means they absorb quickly, a moderate GI (56–69) is slower and a low GI (55 or less) is a slow release.
- GL considers how the quality and quantity of carbs affects blood sugar levels: using a calculation of **(GI × amount of carbs in grams) ÷ 100**, a high GL is 20 or more, medium 11–19 and low 10 or less. Ideally, daily GL should sit under 100.

When it comes to supporting blood sugar levels, try replacing high GI/GL carbohydrates with nutrient-dense, slow releasing low GI/GL carbohydrates. To lower the GI of a food, include it as part of a meal or consume it with a source of protein and/or healthy fats.

Chronic inflammation: A diet high in processed foods and trans fats can lead to chronic inflammation, disrupting hormonal function and potentially leading to conditions like polycystic ovary syndrome (PCOS) in women and hormonal imbalances in men.

Excess weight: Diet plays a pivotal role in maintaining a healthy body weight. Excess body fat, especially around the abdomen, can lead to the overproduction of hormones such as insulin and oestrogen, which is associated with issues including infertility, certain cancers and metabolic disorders.

Hormone-related cancers: Hormone-disrupting chemicals, such as those found in some pesticides and the BPA used in plastic containers, can potentially increase the risk of hormone-related cancers, such as breast, uterine, ovarian and prostate cancer. To protect your hormonal health, choose organic foods and safe food storage practices.

Eating to promote hormonal health

As we've seen, food can help or hinder the natural balance of our hormones, so what we fuel our bodies with matters! An ideal diet is one rich in fibre, antioxidants and anti-inflammatory compounds that support the body's cell function, healthy hormone regulation and natural detoxification processes.

Fruits and vegetables are particularly rich in antioxidants, helping to protect you from harmful compounds and environmental toxins that can disrupt hormonal balance. Try daily juice, as it's a fantastic way to add additional servings to your diet. Lean more towards vegetables than fruit for your base, to keep the fruit sugar, fructose, down.

Healthy drinks

Squeezing the juice of half a lemon or 1 tablespoon of apple cider vinegar into warm water and drinking it each morning will to help stimulate digestive enzymes.

Another drink that helps to support digestion and your liver is dandelion-root coffee, as it increases digestive fluid, enhancing the overall digestive process, including the breakdown of food and absorption of nutrients. Green tea is also beneficial; it contains the bioflavonoid called 'catechin', which is an antioxidant and very healing for the liver.

While caffeine consumption can have a lot of positives, such as improved energy, concentration and its antioxidant properties, if you're sensitive to caffeine it's something to be mindful of, especially when it comes to hormonal health. This is because, being a stimulant, caffeine impacts the nervous system and can increase the circulation of chemicals such as cortisol and adrenaline in the body. This, in turn, can result in feelings of increased anxiety and can even lead to heart palpitations and high blood pressure. Common sources of caffeine include coffee, black tea, green tea, cola drinks, energy drinks and even chocolate. If you are sensitive to the effects of caffeine, opt for decaf coffee, caffeine-free herbal teas such as rooibos, peppermint and chamomile tea and/or dandelion-root coffee, as mentioned above. Eating some food prior to consuming caffeine may assist in lessening its effects, because caffeine is absorbed into the bloodstream more quickly when consumed on an empty stomach.

Herbs and vitamins

Note: It's important to work with your nutritionist, naturopath, dietitian or doctor about recommended doses before taking any supplements.

Liver health

Herbs that can help to improve liver health include globe artichoke, St Mary's thistle, dandelion root, licorice, turmeric, bupleurum, schisandra, astragalus, polygonum, phyllanthus and goldenseal. All of these have a wonderfully stimulating effect on the liver.

The sulphur-containing amino acids methionine, cysteine and taurine, found in sources of protein such as meat, fish, eggs and dairy, help to make detoxifying enzymes in the liver such as glutathione. These enzymes contain antioxidants to protect liver cells and neutralise the effects of drugs and chemicals.

Vitamins B6, B9 and B12 are necessary co-factors in this process. Vitamin C reduces inflammation, fights infection and promotes detoxification, and lecithin can help with fat digestion.

Herbal bitters, such as Swedish bitters – a bitter tonic traditionally used in herbal medicine – can be taken in water before dinner every night. These can be purchased from health food stores and pharmacies.

Adaptogenic herbs

Adaptogenic herbs are herbs and plant substances that support the body to manage stress by interacting with our hypothalamic-pituitary-adrenal axis, which controls our body's stress response. Adaptogenic herbs may be helpful during times of stress to restore balance and build stress tolerance.

DHEA

Dehydroepiandrosterone (DHEA), a steroid hormone produced by the adrenal cortex, is a precursor to other hormones, including testosterone and oestrogen.

Beta-carotene

Beta-carotene is a pigment found in plants such as carrot, sweet potato and green leafy vegetables. Beta-carotene exerts antioxidant activities in the body that assist with overcoming free radical damage and also converts to Vitamin A, which is also an antioxidant, important for eye health, immunity and skin health.

Isoflavones

Isoflavones are polyphenolic compounds and are most abundant in soybeans and legumes. They exert both oestrogenic and/or antioestrogen effects by binding to oestrogen receptors in the body and altering the concentration of endogenous oestrogens. This can make them helpful when managing hormonal conditions such as perimenopause, menopause and postmenopause.

Movement

Train those hormones

Physical activity and movement play an important role in our metabolic function, body composition and mental health. Exercise promotes healthy blood sugar control via increased insulin sensitivity, which can be an effective tool in managing lifestyle diseases such as type 2 diabetes.

Research shows exercise programs can increase appetite-regulating hormones, decrease inflammatory markers and improve lipid profiles and body composition in healthy young men and women. For postmenopausal women, increased exercise can result in weight loss and favourable effects on sex hormones including oestrogens and androgens, which are linked to a decrease in breast cancer risk.

Exercise is also associated with the increased synthesis and release of both neurotransmitters, which are chemical messengers that transmit signals between neurons and influence various physiological process, and neurotrophic factors, which are proteins that support the growth, survival and function of neurons and are crucial for nervous system development and maintenance.

There are so many enjoyable and beneficial activities to choose from, such as dancing, jogging, strength training, swimming or taking a brisk walk with friends. Yoga is a favourite of mine due to its many benefits, so there is a whole section on it below. Variety is the spice of life, and this holds true for exercise as well. Engaging in regular physical activity goes beyond keeping your hormones in check. It's a fantastic way to relax, relieve stress, and spend quality time socialising with friends. The positive impact on your sleep cannot be overstated either, and a good night's rest contributes significantly to hormonal balance.

Yoga

Yoga is an ancient practice that focuses on connection between mind and body using a combination of static poses, gentle movement and breathwork. There are many different types of yoga and it is easy to adjust to different abilities, so it is suitable for people of all ages and fitness levels. Yoga can help to increase strength and flexibility without too much impact on the joints, while reducing stress and blood pressure. I've enlisted some yoga teachers to give examples of how yoga can help to counteract symptoms of changing hormones as we age.

Dr Vibeke Murphy,

holistic chiropractor and yoga teacher

As women transition to perimenopause and menopause, our lean muscle mass decreases. This is because oestrogen has a role in maintenance of lean muscle. When oestrogen levels decrease with advancing perimenopause or menopause, muscle atrophy occurs. Weight-bearing resistance-type yoga poses such as those shown below help to build strength in the muscles and help to maintain lean muscle mass.

Yoga can be a helpful practice during this time to promote physical strength, flexibility and emotional balance. Here's how these asanas can benefit women in perimenopause:

- **Chair Pose:** This pose helps build strength in the legs and spine while also stretching the thoracic area and shoulders. It can enhance balance, which is essential, as hormonal changes can affect coordination.
- **Plank Pose:** Strengthening the core and upper body muscles through plank pose can help maintain overall strength and posture. It's especially beneficial for those dealing with back pain and maintaining good posture during perimenopause.
- **Warrior Two:** This asana helps energise the body and mind while strengthening the legs and opening up the chest and hips. It can help counter feelings of fatigue and sluggishness that can come with hormonal changes.
- **Tree Pose:** Balancing poses like the tree pose are excellent for improving concentration and enhancing overall body strength. Strengthening the vertebral column, thighs and ankle joints can help improve balance and coordination.
- **Cobra Pose:** Cobra pose is beneficial for strengthening the back, which can help alleviate the back pain or discomfort that some women experience during perimenopause. It also stretches and tones the upper back muscles.

It's important to consult a healthcare professional whenever you begin a new physical activity, especially if you have an existing condition or injury. Consider taking classes with experienced instructors who can provide guidance tailored to your stage of life and help you adapt your yoga practice to your specific needs and comfort levels.

Tessa Canny,
Bikram Yoga teacher

The following postures target the rejuvenation and balancing of the endocrine system, for regulation of hormones in the body.

- **Standing Deep-Breathing:** Though not a physical posture, this breathing exercise at the beginning of each Bikram yoga class helps calm the mind and activate the parasympathetic nervous system. It sets the foundation for hormonal balance by reducing stress and promoting relaxation.
- **Half-Moon Pose:** Half-moon pose helps open up the chest and improve circulation, stimulating the thymus gland in the chest, which is involved in the immune system and hormonal regulation.
- **Camel Pose:** Camel pose is a deep backbend that opens up the chest and stretches the entire front of the body. This posture can stimulate the thyroid gland, which is essential for metabolism and hormone regulation.
- **Locust Pose:** Locust pose strengthens the back, glutes and legs; and the compression of the abdomen can stimulate the adrenal glands, which produce hormones like cortisol and adrenaline.
- **Rabbit Pose:** Rabbit pose is a seated forward bend that compresses and stimulates the thyroid gland, helping to balance its function.
- **Cobra Pose:** Cobra pose is a gentle backbend that opens up the chest and stretches the front of the body. It can stimulate the thymus gland, promoting immune function and hormonal balance.
- **Bow Pose:** Bow pose is a backbend that stretches the entire front of the body, stimulating the reproductive organs and supporting hormonal health.
- **Fixed Firm Pose:** Fixed firm pose is a kneeling backbend that stretches the thighs and opens up the hips. It can stimulate the reproductive organs and support hormonal balance.
- **Camel-Rabbit Pose:** This combination pose involves both a backbend (Camel) and a forward bend (Rabbit), providing a balanced compression and stretching of the entire spine. It can have a harmonising effect on the endocrine system.
- **Shoulder Stand:** This pose stimulates the thyroid and parathyroid glands, supporting hormonal regulation.

Marty Cole,
Australian yoga and mindfulness coach and senior facilitator and head of training for Power Living Yoga

- **Wall Squats Sitting on a Block or Chair:** This is a deep squat pose that helps improve hip mobility and flexibility. It can be particularly beneficial for those who have tight hip muscles, as it can aid in loosening the hip joint and increase your range of motion. Improved hip mobility can be beneficial for activities like weightlifting, sports and general flexibility.
- **Sun Salutation A:** Sun Salutation A is a sequence of yoga poses that provide a full-body stretch and promote overall flexibility. It can be a great way to warm up before more intense physical activities or workouts. It also includes a series of deep breaths, which can help with relaxation and focus.
- **Supine Twists:** Twisting poses, such as supine twists, are effective for releasing tension in the spine and hips. These poses can be particularly helpful for those who experience back pain or stiffness, whether due to physical activity, sitting at a desk or other factors.
- **Lunge Twists:** Lunge twists combine dynamic stretching and spinal movement. They can help improve flexibility, balance and stability, making them useful for sports or activities that require agility and quick movements.

These exercises and yoga poses can be valuable in promoting anyone's overall physical and mental wellbeing. The key is to practise these poses safely and with proper alignment, and to choose exercises and stretches that align with your individual fitness goals and needs. It's always a good idea to consult a fitness or yoga professional to ensure that you are performing these exercises correctly and safely.

Mind

Cultivate a healthy mindset

Being in touch with our emotions and grounding ourselves in the 'now' can calm the nervous system, which is intrinsically linked to hormonal health.

When we feel stressed, we produce more 'fight or flight' hormones such as cortisol, adrenaline, dopamine, norepinephrine and epinephrine, to help us escape the threat – real or perceived – that we are facing. While a short burst of stress only has a temporary effect, chronic stress can have a lasting negative impact on our hormones and bodily functions. Chronic stress may decrease thyroid hormone production, leading to thyroid conditions; it can also decrease sex hormone production, which can disrupt menstrual cycles, affect fertility and libido and make the symptoms of perimenopause and menopause worse.

Chronic stress also encourages fat build-up around our tummies and can cause bloating, diarrhoea or constipation due to increased inflammation in the gut. It suppresses the immune system, too, making us more vulnerable to illness, increasing our risk of hypertension, heart attack and stroke.

While acute stress can dampen appetite, chronic stress has a direct impact on our brains' reward and motivation pathways, making us crave highly palatable foods high in fat, sugar and refined carbs, which are low in nutrition and negatively affect blood sugar. There's a link between depression and an increased intake of fast food, snacks and high-energy foods; and a lower intake of vegetables, fruits, lean protein, dairy and grains.

I always encourage my clients to cultivate calmness and grounding practices through things like mantras, meditation and breathing exercises. Listening to relaxing music such as binaural beats and isochronic tones, which are assistant forms of meditation using pulses of sound that help calm the mind, can also be beneficial. These techniques help them to engage in mindfulness, find balance, create centredness and reduce stress.

The importance of sleep cannot be underestimated in supporting wellness of the mind. In all life stages, consistent, quality sleep is crucial for hormonal balance, cognitive function, emotional wellbeing and overall health. Developing and maintaining healthy sleep habits can positively impact hormonal regulation and contribute to a healthier and more balanced life. I always emphasise healthy sleep hygiene with my clients, which is not just about getting enough sleep each night but putting into practice good pre-bedtime habits. Good sleep hygiene can include avoiding stimulants too close to bedtime, not going to bed hungry or too full, curtailing screen time and dimming the lights at least an hour before bed, and using tools such as meditation or calming music to relax.

Practise positivity

There are so many brilliant tools to help you live a positive and less stressful life. Keeping a gratitude journal encourages a positive mindset, while mindfulness apps aid in staying present and reducing anxiety. Listening to calming music lowers stress levels, and limiting screen time, especially before bedtime, improves sleep quality. Adequate sleep positively impacts mood and overall functioning. Saunas contribute to stress reduction through relaxation and detoxification. Repeating mantras, especially positive and personal affirmations that reflect the goals and intentions you're trying to focus on, can very centring and calming.

Meditation is a very powerful tool, but if you're new to meditation, start with short sessions and gradually extend the duration as you become more comfortable. Find a quiet space, sit or lie comfortably and focus on your breath or use guided meditation apps to assist you. Experiment with different types of meditation, such as mindfulness or loving-kindness meditation, to discover what resonates with you. There are so many free apps and online resources for you to play around with and find what works best for you. Consistency is key, so aim for regular but manageable sessions.

Seeking professional help can also be hugely beneficial to fostering a positive relationship with yourself. When it comes to finding a counsellor or therapist, in my experience it's such a personal exercise and it's important to consider your specific needs. I find asking for recommendations from friends, family, or your healthcare practitioner can be very helpful. Online directories and mental health organisations are also valuable resources. A good fit with your therapist is important, so don't hesitate to book an initial consultation to see if your personalities and goals are aligned.

Remember, working on your inner narrative, developing a positive mindset and expressing gratitude can not only benefit your mental health, but also affect your ability to make diet and lifestyle choices supportive of hormonal health.

Breathe

How you breathe has a profound impact on your health and wellbeing. I often recommend that my clients try breathing exercises as a way of grounding themselves and releasing stress. I'm going to share a few simple examples with you: box breathing, triangle breathing, 2-to-1 breathing and alternate nostril breathing. To help me, I've called on an expert, Sari Shillingford – an XPT-certified Breathwork teacher, meditation facilitator and Pilates instructor. The deep breathing exercises that Sari recommends have been positively associated with everything from better sleep and improved heart health to improved digestion, reduced anxiety and depression and enhanced cognitive function.

You can do these breathing exercises anywhere, without any equipment. All you need is time, attention and a bit of practice.

Box breathing

Box breathing is a powerful but simple relaxation technique that involves four basic steps, each of equal length: inhale, hold, exhale and hold.

It is easy to do, quick to learn and can be highly effective in stressful situations to return breathing to its natural rhythm. This technique is also relevant for anyone interested in re-centring themselves or improving their concentration and focus while flooding the body with a wave of relaxation.

You can count to any number you choose during each of these parts, although I'm suggesting a 4 count below. As the name implies, the pattern of breathing can be symbolised by a box.

You can practise box breathing for 5–10 cycles or several minutes at a time, as often as needed. The breathwork is practised through the nostrils with the mouth closed.

To practise box breathing:

- Sit comfortably, with your spine upright and your back supported, either with your legs crossed or, if seated on a chair, your feet flat on the ground with your hands resting in your lap.
- Focus on keeping your breath moving into your belly, slow, smooth and continuous.
- Inhale for a count of 4.
- Hold for a count of 4.
- Exhale for a count of 4.
- Hold for a count of 4.
- Repeat.

Triangle breathing

Triangle breathing is a simple relaxation technique that involves three basic steps, each of equal length: inhale, hold, exhale.

It is easy to do, quick to learn and can be highly effective in stressful situations to return breathing to its natural rhythm. This technique is also relevant for anyone interested in re-centring themselves or improving their concentration and focus while flooding the body with a wave of relaxation.

You can count to any number you choose during each of these parts, although I'm suggesting a 4 count below. As the name implies, the pattern of breathing can be symbolised by a triangle.

You can practise triangle breathing for 5–10 cycles or several minutes at a time, as often as needed. The breathwork is practised through the nostrils with the mouth closed.

To practise triangle breathing:

- Sit comfortably, with your spine upright and your back supported, either with your legs crossed or, if seated on a chair, your feet flat on the ground with your hands resting in your lap.
- Focus on keeping your breath moving into your belly, slow, smooth and continuous.
- Start at the bottom corner of the inverted triangle.
- Inhale for a count of 4.
- Hold for a count of 4.
- Exhale for a count of 4.
- Repeat.

2-to-1 breathing

2-to-1 breathing is a powerful technique that involves two basic steps: inhale, then exhale for twice the duration of your inhalation.

This technique can help us restore inner balance, assist in overcoming nervousness and ignite creativity. It is an effective way to calm the nervous system and prepare the body and mind for meditation and/or sleep.

You can practise 2-to-1 breathing for 5–10 cycles or several minutes at a time, as often as needed.

You can count to any number you choose during these parts, although I'm suggesting an inhale for 3 counts and an exhale for 6 counts below.

Focus on your breath as your heart rate slows, your blood pressure drops and your muscles begin to relax.

To practise 2-to-1 breathing:

- Sit comfortably, with your spine upright and your back supported, either with your legs crossed or, if seated on a chair, your feet flat on the ground with your hands resting in your lap.
- Focus on keeping your breath slow, smooth and continuous.
- Close your mouth and breathe lightly through your nose.
- Start to adjust your breathing – focus on keeping your breath moving into your belly, slow, smooth and continuous.
- Inhale for a count of 3.
- Exhale for a count of 6.
- Repeat.

Alternate nostril breathing

Alternate nostril breathing offers a host of benefits: it triggers a relaxation response, helps ease stress and anxiety, improves brain function and leaves you feeling balanced and ready for dynamic activity or deep rest.

You can practise alternate nostril breathing for 5–10 cycles or several minutes at a time, as often as needed.

As you advance in your practice, you can gradually increase the length of your breaths.

Always end by exhaling through your left nostril.

To practise alternate nostril breathing:

- Sit comfortably, with your spine upright and your back supported, either with your legs crossed or, if seated on a chair, your feet flat on the ground with your left hand resting on your left knee.
- Focus on keeping your breath slow, smooth and continuous.
- Lift your right hand up to your nose.
- Exhale completely, then use your right thumb to close your right nostril.
- Inhale through your left nostril, then close it with your pointer finger.
- Open your right nostril and exhale through it.
- Inhale through your right nostril, then close it with your thumb.
- Open your left nostril and exhale through it.
- Repeat.

Connection

Find your tribe

Many people tend to feel more secure when they know that they have others around them who support their goals and care about their progress. A simple connection between people (such as shared goals or interests) is enough to increase feelings of warmth and motivation; and ultimately, people seem wired to adopt the goals of the people around them, which also promotes stress reduction and an increase of 'happy' neurochemicals and positive hormonal health.

Studies have identified numerous positive effects of having a healthy sense of belonging, including more positive social relationships, academic achievement, occupational success and better physical and mental health. A lack of belonging, in turn, has been linked to an increased risk for mental and physical health problems.

Conventional Medicine

Follow the science

Conventional medicine, also known as western medicine or mainstream medicine, is a science-backed approach that doctors and other healthcare professionals such as nurses, therapists and pharmacists use to diagnose and treat symptoms and conditions.

Conventional medicine can help not only with symptom control but also long-term management and treatment of underlying conditions affecting hormonal health.

Diet and nutrition medicine is a medical field focusing on the role that nutrition plays in health, disease, lifecycle and ageing. Like other forms of conventional medicine, it seeks to address the underlying cause of a person's symptoms where possible, not merely trying to manage them but also promoting inner body balance.

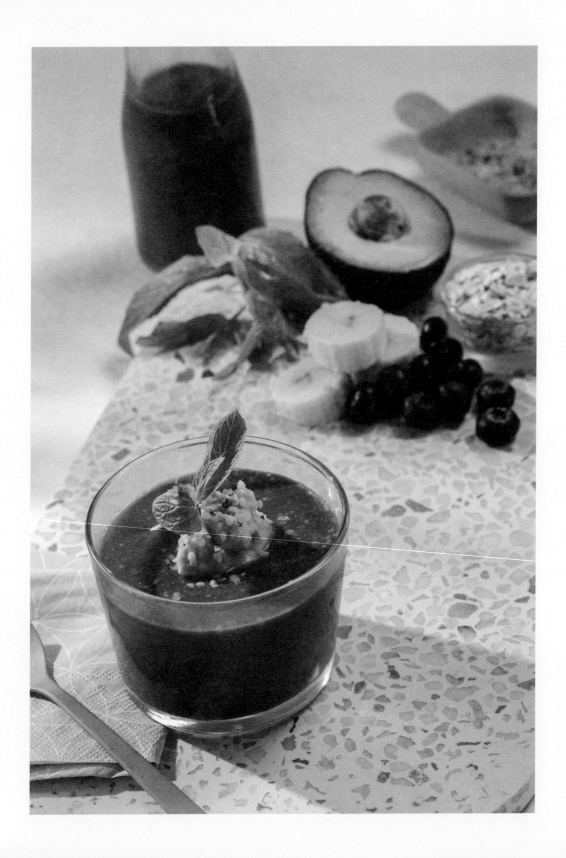

Hormone Specifics

Hormones and Thyroid Health

Support your thyroid function

The thyroid is a small, butterfly-shaped gland at the front of the neck. It produces the hormones thyroxine (T4), triiodothyronine (T3) and calcitonin. T4 and T3 are important for metabolism, heart rate and body temperature, while calcitonin controls the levels of calcium and phosphate in the blood. In turn, thyroid hormones have an effect on virtually every system in the body including the nervous system, cardiovascular system, musculoskeletal system, gastrointestinal system and reproductive system.

If your body produces too much or too little T4 and/or T3 , you can experience a whole range of debilitating symptoms, which in rare cases, if left untreated, can be life-threatening. From a reproductive perspective, thyroid conditions can negatively impact fertility and reproductive system function generally. Thankfully, thyroid conditions can easily be managed with medication, supplements and dietary and lifestyle changes, once diagnosed.

Research has shown that women, older people and those with a family history of thyroid disease are most at risk of thyroid disease.

Hypothyroidism

An underactive thyroid leads to thyroid hormone deficiency. Its primary causes are iodine deficiency, radiation, surgery, prescription and illicit drugs (drug-induced hypothyroidism) and autoimmune disorders, such as Hashimoto's disease, in which the immune system attacks the thyroid gland, causing it to become inflamed and unable to make sufficient thyroid hormones. The most common secondary cause is hypopituitarism, a rare condition where the pituitary gland does not make adequate hormones. The thyroid gland won't work properly if it doesn't receive adequate hormones from the pituitary gland.

Symptoms of an underactive thyroid include weight gain, difficulty tolerating cold, fatigue, mood changes, impaired memory, constipation, infertility, dry hair, hair loss and low libido.

Hyperthyroidism

An overactive thyroid leads to an oversupply of thyroid hormones. The most common condition associated with hyperthyroidism is the autoimmune disorder Graves' disease. Like Hashimoto's disease, Graves' disease attacks the thyroid, but in this case it has the opposite effect, causing it to make an excessive amount of thyroid hormone. Hyperthyroidism can also present temporarily after a virus due to inflammation of the thyroid gland causing excess production of thyroid hormone. Symptoms of an overactive thyroid include weight loss, increased appetite, a rapid or irregular heartbeat, nervousness, irritability, shaky hands, sweating, trouble sleeping and frequent bowel movements.

Sex, stress and thyroid function

The interaction between thyroid hormones and other hormones your body produces is also significant. Sex hormones and stress hormones deserve special mention here.

Sex hormones: When oestrogen, progesterone or other sex hormones are out of balance, it can affect the functioning of thyroid hormones. For example, elevated oestrogen can trigger an increase in the production of thyroid binding globulin (TBG), which binds to thyroid hormones and decreases the amount available for use by the body, leading to symptoms of hypothyroidism. In such cases, correcting underlying sex hormone imbalances may help to balance thyroid function.

Stress hormones: Stress-induced cortisol production can also affect the thyroid, especially over the long term. High levels of cortisol in our system tell the thyroid that our survival is under threat, and it responds by producing a mirror image of T3, called reverse T3 (RT3). RT3 is the body's shutdown signal: it says to the body there are not enough resources to sustain all biological functions of the body so non-essential functions, such as reproduction, must be shut down to reserve resources for essential functions, like those of the heart, kidneys and other organs keeping us alive. To overcome this, it's important to reduce stress hormone production, to blunt the production of RT3 and repair normal thyroid function.

Diagnosis

To check your thyroid function, your doctor will order blood tests. High TSH and low T4 are indicative of hypothyroidism. Low TSH and high T3 and T4 are indicative of hyperthyroidism. If your doctor suspects an autoimmune disorder, like Hashimoto's or Graves' disease, they will test for the presence of thyroid antibodies. In an autoimmune thyroid disorder, rogue antibodies are created by the immune system and they mistakenly target the thyroid gland, leading to inflammation, tissue damage and/or poor thyroid function.

The symptoms of thyroid imbalance can mimic those of perimenopause, often leading to confusion in diagnosis. A blood test is an easy way to check what's going on if you have any doubt.

Eating to support thyroid function

The choices you make when you're selecting foods, planning meals and cooking can do a lot to help keep thyroid hormones in balance. For example, certain foods such as raw cruciferous vegetables and soy products contain compounds called goitrogens, which can interfere with thyroid hormone production. While these foods are incredibly healthy generally, they may be something to be mindful of when trying to support or overcome a thyroid condition.

Remember that individual dietary needs and thyroid conditions can vary, and certain foods and supplements can impact thyroid medication absorption, so it's crucial to consult a suitably qualified healthcare provider, registered nutritionist or dietitian for personalised advice on managing thyroid health. They can help you make dietary choices that align with your specific health needs and goals.

Underactive thyroid

To support a sluggish thyroid, you can:

- **Check your iodine levels.** A blood or urine test will tell you if you're getting enough iodine, which is important for thyroid hormone production. Foods high in iodine include asparagus, cod, dairy, iodised salt, oysters and seaweed.
- **Check your iron levels.** Iron deficiency makes the thyroid less responsive to iodine. Foods high in iron include red meat, liver, almonds, apricots, sunflower seeds and pumpkin seeds.
- **Eat foods rich in zinc and selenium.** You need zinc and selenium to convert T4 to T3. Foods high in zinc include beef, capsicum, eggs and

pumpkin seeds. Foods high in selenium include barley, brazil nuts, broccoli, cashews, peanuts, and tuna.

- **Eat foods rich in tyrosine.** You need tyrosine, an amino acid, to make thyroid hormones. Foods high in tyrosine include almonds, avocado, bananas, beef, cheese, chicken, eggs, fish and whey protein.
- **Make sure you're getting enough carbs.** Too few carbohydrates can affect the production of T3. Make complex, fibre-rich carbs such as whole grains, brown rice, sourdough bread, root veggies, quinoa, freekeh and legumes a regular part of your diet. Pair carbs with protein and healthy fats to support healthy blood sugar levels.
- **Cook your cruciferous veggies.** When they're raw, broccoli, cabbage, cauliflower, kale and other cruciferous vegetables contain goitrogens. Cook these veggies instead of eating them raw, and don't eat too much of them, especially if your iodine levels are low.
- **Cut back on soy.** Soy also contains goitrogens, so steer clear of tofu, tempeh, edamame and soy milk.
- **Cut back on inflammatory foods.** Inflammation is correlated with low thyroid function, so try to stay away from processed meats, refined sugar, refined oils and too much omega-6 vs omega-3. Omega-6 fats are known to be pro-inflammatory, whereas omega-3 fats are anti-inflammatory.

Overactive thyroid

To rein in an overactive thyroid, you can:

- **Cut back on iodine and tyrosine.** Thyroid hormones are made from iodine and tyrosine. If you already have an overactive thyroid and eat foods high in iodine and tyrosine, your body will produce even more T4, making the situation even worse.
- **Eat foods rich in antioxidants.** Hyperthyroidism is known to cause increased oxidative stress, a disruption between the production of free radicals and antioxidant defences. Consuming a diet high in antioxidants may assist with addressing this. Food high in antioxidants include berries, brightly coloured veggies, leafy greens and herbs.
- **Eat foods rich in zinc and selenium.** As noted above, you need zinc and selenium to convert T4 to T3. Foods high in zinc include beef, capsicum, eggs, and pumpkin seeds. Foods high in selenium include barley, brazil nuts, broccoli, cashews, peanuts and tuna.

Hormones and Liver Health

Support your liver function

A t one time or another, we've all eaten the wrong things, had too much to drink, celebrated too hard or slept too little. If you're in this situation, I'd recommend you try an internal cleanse. It's comforting to know that our body is *always* detoxing, thanks to our trusty liver, but after placing excess pressure on any one part of our body, we really should give it a break, to help it regain some natural balance. This is exactly what detoxing is all about.

A healthy liver is as important as a healthy brain for optimal health. So, let's look at what can happen when we indulge in all those silly season antics that are fun at the time but not so fun for our bodies afterwards.

How the liver works

The liver plays a crucial role in hormone metabolism, processing and clearing hormones from the bloodstream. There are two primary pathways through which the liver helps with hormone regulation: the synthesis and clearance of hormones.

Hormone synthesis: The liver is involved in the synthesis of some hormones, especially those related to lipid metabolism. For example, it synthesises insulin-like growth factor 1 (IGF-1), which supports cell growth and repair. Additionally, the liver is responsible for producing certain proteins that bind to hormones and carry them through the bloodstream. One such protein is sex hormone–binding globulin (SHBG), which binds to sex hormones like testosterone and oestrogen, regulating their distribution and availability in the body.

Hormone clearance: After hormones have done their work, they need to be cleared from the bloodstream to prevent hormonal imbalances. The liver processes and breaks down these hormones, making them less active and easier for the body to eliminate. This process occurs through two main pathways: conjugation and excretion. Conjugation involves adding a molecule to the hormone, making it water-soluble and easier to eliminate. The liver then excretes these conjugated hormones into the bile, which eventually reaches the intestines. From there, they are excreted from the body through faeces. Some hormones are also secreted directly into the urine.

Detoxification is a metabolic process whereby not-so-friendly substances, for example alcohol and pesticides, are changed into more 'friendly' substances in preparation for their excretion from the body.

Excess and metabolic hormones need to be removed from the body; otherwise, if they are recirculated, it can lead to and compound hormonal imbalances. This means, from a hormonal perspective, healthy detoxification is important.

In a nutshell, detoxification occurs over a few phases:

Phase 1: A group of enzymes called cytochrome P450 and specific vitamins and minerals transform dangerous substances into less harmful substances through chemical processes.

Phase 2: A chemical group is added to the metabolites formed in phase 1, to make them water soluble and easier to transport and eliminate.

Phase 3: The phase 2 substances are eliminated, mostly via urine and bowel movements.

Signs that the detox pathways are sluggish include:
- nausea and lack of appetite, especially upon waking
- bloating and poor digestion
- constipation or sluggish bowels
- poor tolerance of fatty foods, caffeine and alcohol
- inability to lose weight, or recent weight gain
- fatigue, lack of vitality and feelings of irritability
- more frequent skin breakouts and dull skin tone
- grey rings around the eyes
- poor sleep or disrupted sleep.

Nutritional imbalances also affect the healthy bacteria contained in the gut. The result is referred to as 'dysbiosis', and it can often cause inflammation of the digestive tract, as well as bacterial, fungal or parasitic infection, or intestinal permeability. If the gut wall then becomes weakened, additional protein can leak into the bloodstream and initiate allergic reactions. Then the liver's ability to detoxify the body is threatened. Fatigue, weight gain and poor skin are common symptoms of these digestive and liver overload problems.

Liver overload

The symptoms of liver overload include aching muscles, loss of appetite, bloating, nausea, jaundice (turning yellow, including the whites of the eyes), diarrhoea, dark-coloured urine, abdominal discomfort, tiredness, light-coloured stools, irritability, itching and flu-like symptoms.

The good news is that these symptoms can be addressed through improved nutrition. Specific nutrients can help enhance your liver function, including antioxidants (found in foods rich in vitamins A, C, E, coenzyme Q10 and zinc), amino acids and phytochemicals (glucosinolates, which are found in vegetables such as brussels sprouts).

Following a detoxification diet is another way to help your liver recover from overload.

Detoxing

Detoxing is something that should be done for a minimum of five days, and, depending on how toxic you are feeling, a maximum of a month. This is partly for your body and partly for your sanity!

While you are detoxing, you may experience headaches, nausea or energy lows. If you do experience any of these symptoms, remember that they won't last forever and are a natural effect of detoxing. Keep going – they will only last a couple of days, and once you are through them you will feel fantastic!

After you have followed a detoxification diet, you will find that your energy levels have increased or are more even throughout the day. Your digestive system will be noticeably better, with fewer irritable bowel movements and less bloating.

The key to successful detoxing is eliminating foods and liquids that are toxic to the body or that place extra pressure on the liver.

Food and drink to avoid

- alcohol
- dairy products
- caffeine drinks, such as coffee, tea or cola
- refined sugars, such as white table sugar
- saturated fats or trans fats, including fried foods, animal fats, heated oils, margarines and spreadable butters)

- red meat, and chicken with skin
- refined flour products (including breads, cakes, biscuits and all baked goods)
- processed foods
- tinned, and bottled foods
- 'fat-free' foods
- foods containing preservatives, colouring or additives

Foods to eat

- legumes and pulses (including adzuki beans, dry peas, lentils, soybeans, kidney beans, chickpeas, black beans and broad beans)
- unprocessed grains (including brown rice, buckwheat, quinoa, amaranth, barley, oats, corn, rye and millet)
- good fats, such as essential fatty acids
- raw, unsalted seeds and nuts
- avocados
- extra-virgin olive oil, flaxseed oil and oily fish (all in small portions)
- lean red meat and chicken without skin (150-gram serves, no more than once daily)
- pineapple, lemons, grapefruit, pears, grapes, artichokes, shiitake mushrooms, garlic, carrot, beetroot, cucumber and bitter lettuce, such as rocket and chicory

Beverages to drink

- filtered water
- warm water with lemon or apple cider vinegar
- dandelion-root coffee
- fresh vegetable juices
- coconut kefir
- kombucha
- green tea

Optional: herbs and supplements

- globe artichoke, St Mary's thistle, dandelion root, licorice, turmeric, bupleurum, schisandra, astragalus, polygonum, phyllanthus and goldenseal
- glutathione
- vitamin B complex
- vitamin C lecithin
- herbal bitters, such as Swedish bitters

Sample detox day

Pre-breakfast: Lemon juice in hot water and fresh vegetable juice

Breakfast: Fruit salad with soy or rice yoghurt and 1 tablespoon of raw nuts and seeds

Snack: A peach and a handful of mixed nuts

Lunch: Organic or free-range grilled or oven baked chicken breast marinated in extra-virgin olive oil, lemon juice, sea salt with a mixed salad, avocado, tomato dressed with lemon juice, olive oil and herbs

Snack: A small smoothie made of fruit and soy, rice, oat or almond milk

Dinner: Vegetable, beans and lentil soup

Post-dinner: Herbal tea with fruit and nuts

Hormones and Iron

The best foods for increasing iron levels

Iron is an important mineral that helps to transport oxygen around the body; it also plays a role in many bodily functions, including immunity. In fact, iron is known as the 'energy mineral', because when we are low in iron, common symptoms are fatigue and feelings of sluggishness. Iron levels can be checked via a blood test.

One of the best ways to maintain healthy iron levels is to consume adequate iron in our diets. Dietary iron is classified as haem iron (from animal sources) or non-haem iron (from plant sources), with haem iron being the more absorbable form.

Iron is particularly important for women due to their unique physiological and reproductive needs.

As we know, women of childbearing age experience monthly menstrual periods, during which they lose blood. This loss can lead to iron deficiency over time if iron is not adequately replenished. Iron is a key component of haemoglobin, the protein in red blood cells that carries oxygen to tissues and organs. Insufficient iron can result in anaemia, leading to fatigue, weakness and reduced energy levels.

Throughout pregnancy, iron needs increase to support the growth and development of the foetus. Adequate iron intake is essential for preventing iron-deficiency anaemia in pregnant women, as well as ensuring a healthy birth weight for the baby.

After childbirth, women may experience blood loss, which further depletes iron stores. Adequate iron intake during the postpartum period is important for recovery and healing.

Breastfeeding mothers have increased iron needs to support both their own health and the nutritional needs of their infants. Iron is passed from the mother's milk to the baby, and ensuring sufficient iron levels is crucial for the baby's growth and development.

Many women, especially vegetarians and vegans, may have a low intake of haem iron. This can make it more challenging to meet daily iron requirements, so careful attention to iron-rich plant-based foods is important.

Some women experience heavier menstrual bleeding than average, a condition known as menorrhagia. This can lead to increased iron loss and a higher risk of iron-deficiency anaemia. Adequate iron intake is essential to counteract these effects.

Iron also plays a role in maintaining bone health, which is especially significant for women as they are more prone than men to conditions like osteoporosis. Iron contributes to collagen formation, a key component of bone structure.

Iron is vital for overall energy levels and cognitive function. Iron deficiency can lead to fatigue, weakness and reduced mental alertness, affecting a woman's daily life and productivity.

How much iron do we need?

The recommended dietary intake (RDI) of iron per day varies depending on age, gender and other factors such as pregnancy. The current RDIs are outlined in the below tables.

Children

Boys & Girls

Age (years)	RDI (day)
1–3	9 mg
4–8	10 mg

Adolescents

Boys

Age (years)	RDI (day)
9–13	8 mg
14–18	11 mg

Girls

Age (years)	RDI (day)
9–13	8 mg
14–18	15 mg

Adults

Men

Age (years)	RDI (day)
19+	8 mg

Women

Age (years)	RDI (day)
19–50	18 mg
51+	8 mg
pregnant women	27 mg

Source: Nutrient Reference Values for Australia and New Zealand

So, which foods contain iron?

Here are some examples of foods containing haem and non-haem iron with their approximate iron content. Note: These measurements are based on raw weights unless otherwise specified.

Haem (animal)

- chicken liver 100 g = 9.80 mg
- octopus 100 g = 5.30 mg
- oyster 100 g = 3.47 mg
- kangaroo 100 g = 3.40 mg
- beef 100 g = 1.30 mg
- squid 100 g = 1.30 mg
- tuna (canned) 100 g = 1.16 mg
- salmon (canned) 100 g = 1.14 mg
- egg × 1 = 0.84 mg
- veal 100 g = 0.58 mg
- lamb 100 g = 0.41 mg
- white fish 100 g = 0.40 mg
- salmon 100 g = 0.31 mg
- chicken breast 100 g = 0.26 mg

Non-haem (plant)

- chia seeds 100 g = 13.00 mg
- pumpkin seeds 100 g = 8.50 mg
- tahini 100 mL = 5.10 mg
- cashews 100 g = 5.00 mg
- sunflower seeds 100 g = 4.85 mg
- wholemeal pasta 100 g = 3.90 mg
- almonds 100 g = 3.75 mg
- oats 100 g = 3.50 mg
- apricots (dried) 100 g = 3.10 mg
- tofu (firm) 100 g = 2.35 mg
- red kidney beans (boiled) 100 g = 2.19 mg
- wholemeal bread 100 g = 1.97 mg

- chickpeas (boiled) 100 g = 1.80 mg
- spinach 100 g = 1.75 mg
- lentils (boiled) 100 g = 1.63 mg
- kale 100 g = 1.60 mg
- figs (dried) 100 g = 1.40 mg
- prunes (dried) 100 g = 1.10 mg
- rye sourdough bread 100 g = 1.10 mg
- broccoli 100 g = 0.84 mg

Source: Australian Foods Composition Database

Iron fortified foods

Foods fortified with iron (i.e. foods that iron has been added to) can be used to help increase iron intake. There are many on the market, including:

- cereals, offering around 3 mg iron per serve (6.70 mg per 100 g)
- bread, which offers around 4 mg iron per serve (6.00 mg per 100 g).

Iron inhibitors

Be mindful of iron inhibitors – these are compounds found in foods which, depending on their quantity, can inhibit mostly non-haem iron absorption.
In order to maximise iron absorption, it is best to avoid too much of the below foods when consuming iron-rich foods:

- Foods rich in polyphenols, including tannins, such as red wine, cocoa, tea and coffee. (It's best to drink tea and coffee etc a few hours away from meals.)
- Phytates – found in whole grains (e.g. wheat bran, wheatgerm, rice bran and sorghum), nuts and seeds (e.g. linseeds, sesame seeds, sunflower seeds, almonds, walnuts and cashews) and legumes (e.g. red kidney beans, soy beans, chickpeas and lentils).
- Calcium – found in dairy products (e.g milk, yoghurt and cheese). Calcium supplements have also been shown to have an impact on both haem and non-haem iron.

Iron tips and tricks to aid intake and absorption

There are some known ways to enhance iron absorption, especially non-haem iron, including:

- Consuming non-haem sources of iron with foods rich in ascorbic acid (vitamin C) – e.g. berries, capsicum, tomatoes, cauliflower, papaya and parsley.
- Consuming non-haem sources of iron with foods rich in lactic acid – e.g. sourdough bread, fermented foods and pickled veggies.
- Consuming both haem and non-haem sources of iron together can also increase absorption from plant foods. For example, serve fish or meat with a legume salad, or fish or meat on top of a chickpea curry.
- Cooking plant foods rich in non-haem iron (e.g. leafy greens) can increase the amount of available iron.
- Soaking and sprouting legumes, pulses, grains and seeds can help to reduce phytate levels.
- If supplementing with iron, it can be taken every second day, as it will stay in the system for a couple of days. Also, it's best taken on an empty stomach.

With the above in mind, here are some practical tips to help with both iron intake and absorption:

- Add strawberries/berries and hemp seeds to fortified cereal or oats in the morning.
- Use orange juice when making Bircher muesli and top with berries.
- Serve eggs on toast with a side of cooked spinach and tomatoes or fresh fruit.
- Add lemon/lime juice to salad dressings.
- Choose veggies rich in vitamin C, such as tomato, capsicum, broccoli and cauliflower, for salads, wraps and sandwiches.
- Swap regular bread for sourdough.
- Add a spoonful of fermented veggies to main meals.
- Add some raw veggies and fruit to your diet.
- Avoid overcooking veggies, as vitamin C is quite susceptible to loss when exposed to heat.
- If you aren't a big meat fan, try replacing half a portion of meat with half a portion of legumes when making dishes.
- Mash beans or chickpeas and use them as a sandwich/wrap/toast spread.

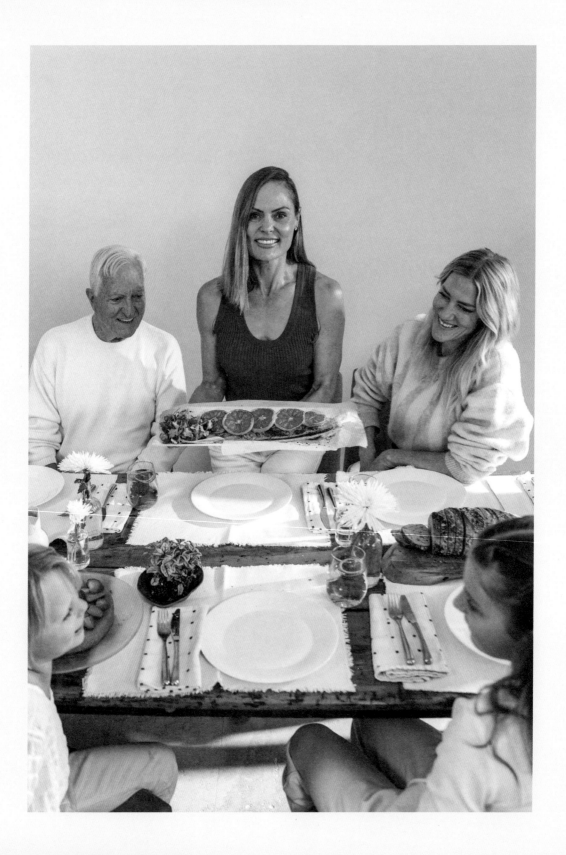

The Hormonal Stages

Tweens

As the mother of an energetic nine-year-old girl, I know only too well the warp and weft of the intricate tapestry of her development. For almost a decade, I have watched her blossom: from a happy and contented baby into an adventurous toddler, filled with curiosity about the world around her, and then the active, school-aged child she is now, who loves netball, karate and long summer days at the beach.

The evolving fabric of my daughter's physical, mental, emotional and social expressions as she has gone through each developmental stage has been magical to observe and even more amazing to nurture ... and it's even more amazing now, as she enters her tween years.

While hormones play a part in our childhood development, they become much more significant as we enter puberty, typically starting around ages 9 to 11.

The tween years, broadly spanning the ages of 9 to 12, are a bridge between the innocence of childhood and the complexities of adolescence. It is during this time that the body's endocrine system undergoes hormonal shifts, triggering remarkable transformations that lay the foundation for the next phase of life.

Sleep is crucial at all stages and during puberty, growth hormone is released during deep sleep, promoting physical development and supporting the changes that come with adolescence. A good night's sleep helps support emotional and appetite regulation and helps maintain focus.

Both girls and boys often want more independence at this age, as they try to make sense of the changes they're going through as puberty begins. Girls may develop breast tissue and even have their first menstrual cycle during this phase. Similarly, boys may experience an increase in testicle size, pubic hair development and a growth spurt.

Several hormones play pivotal roles in these physical and emotional changes. They include:

- **Growth Hormone (GH):** As its name suggests, growth hormone is responsible for growth. It stimulates the development of bones and tissues, leading to the growth spurts that often occur during the tween years. This hormone is instrumental in a child's physical development during this phase.
- **Gonadotropin-Releasing Hormone (GnRH):** This hormone brings on the beginning of puberty. It triggers the release of other hormones by the pituitary gland, which in turn trigger the development of primary and secondary sexual characteristics.
- **Follicle-Stimulating Hormone (FSH) and Luteinising Hormone (LH):** These hormones are released by the pituitary gland in response to GnRH. In girls, FSH and LH stimulate the ovaries to produce oestrogen, initiating the menstrual cycle. In boys, they stimulate the testes to produce testosterone.
- **Oestrogen:** Oestrogen is the primary sex hormone in females. During the tween years, girls experience a gradual increase in oestrogen levels, which triggers the development of secondary sexual characteristics like breast development and the widening of hips. Oestrogen also plays a role in regulating the menstrual cycle.
- **Testosterone:** Testosterone is the primary sex hormone in males. It's responsible for the development of male secondary sexual characteristics such as facial hair growth, deepening of the voice and muscle development. During the tween years, boys experience an increase in testosterone levels, triggering these changes.
- **Adrenocorticotropic Hormone (ACTH) and Cortisol:** These hormones play a role in managing stress and regulating metabolism. Their levels can fluctuate during the tween years, potentially impacting mood and energy levels.
- **Insulin:** While not a sex hormone, insulin's role in regulating blood sugar becomes increasingly important as the body grows and changes. Changes in insulin sensitivity can occur during the tween years, potentially increasing the risk of developing conditions like type 2 diabetes.

These hormones collectively bring about the myriad changes that occur during the tween years, setting the stage for the transition from childhood to adolescence. The interactions between these hormones and genetic and environmental factors contribute to the unique experiences and developmental paths of the individual child.

Nutrition is key to this, so what foods should the tween in our life be eating to support their hormonal growth?

Hormone Supportive Foods

These foods are beneficial for supporting tweens' health and hormonal balance due to their nutrient profiles and various health-promoting properties:

- **Hemp Seeds:** Hemp seeds are rich in vital fatty acids, particularly omega-3 and omega-6, which are crucial for hormonal balance. They also provide protein and minerals, supporting overall growth and development during the tween years.
- **Nuts:** Nuts offer healthy fats, vitamins and minerals that are essential for the production and regulation of hormones. They provide a convenient and nutritious snack for tweens.
- **Avocado:** Avocado is a source of monounsaturated fats, which play a role in hormone production and overall health. It also provides vitamins and minerals important for growth and development.
- **Salmon and Tuna:** Fatty fish like salmon and tuna are rich in omega-3 fatty acids, which support hormonal balance and reduce inflammation. These fish also offer high-quality protein, needed for growth and repair.
- **Chicken:** Lean poultry like chicken is a good source of protein, essential for muscle development and growth. It also contains B vitamins, which aid in energy metabolism.
- **Whole Grains:** Whole grains like brown rice, quinoa, buckwheat and oats supply complex carbohydrates and fibre, promoting stable blood sugar levels and hormonal balance. They provide sustained energy for tweens.
- **Leafy Greens:** Leafy greens such as spinach and kale are packed with vitamins, minerals and antioxidants that support overall health and hormonal regulation.
- **Legumes and Pulses:** Legumes and pulses, including beans and lentils, are rich in plant-based protein, fibre and various vitamins and minerals. They contribute to sustained energy levels and support growth.
- **Red Meat:** Red meat, such as lean beef, provides iron, zinc and protein. These nutrients are crucial for preventing anaemia and supporting growth, especially during the tween years.
- **Seafood:** Seafood, besides being a source of omega-3 fatty acids, offers minerals like iodine, which is vital for thyroid hormone production and regulation.
- **Pumpkin Seeds:** Pumpkin seeds are high in zinc, a mineral that plays a role in hormone production and immune function. They also provide healthy fats and protein.

- **Chia Seeds:** Chia seeds are a source of omega-3 fatty acids, fibre and antioxidants, supporting digestion and providing vital nutrients for hormonal balance.
- **Natural Yoghurt:** Natural yoghurt contains probiotics that promote gut health. A healthy gut microbiome can indirectly influence hormonal balance and overall wellbeing.
- **Kefir:** Similar to yoghurt, kefir is a probiotic-rich fermented milk drink that supports gut health and may positively impact hormonal regulation.
- **Fruits:** Fruits of all kinds are rich in vitamins, minerals, antioxidants and fibre. They contribute to overall health and can help maintain stable blood sugar levels.

Including a balanced combination of these foods in a tween's diet can provide them with the essential nutrients needed to support healthy growth and hormonal balance during this important stage of development.

Key foods for your tweens

Kids need proper nutrition, not only to help them physically get through the school day but also to focus well in class, so paying close attention to what goes into their meals at home and at school is one of the best gifts you can give them.

Preparing healthy food for your tween can be a real struggle, though! To lend a helping hand, I have outlined below the main nutrients they need. I've included examples of foods rich in these nutrients and some simple suggestions for including them in lunch boxes in kid-friendly ways.

Protein

Food sources of protein supply amino acids, which the body uses for growth, development and muscle repair. Protein also makes you feel full, which helps to stabilise blood sugar levels and therefore supports energy levels.

Example food sources: eggs, fish, meat, dairy (milk, cheese, yoghurt), nuts/seeds, tofu, and legumes and pulses.

Using protein in meals/snacks:

- Use eggs, fish, meat or cheese in wraps or sandwiches.
- Use crumbled tofu or scrambled eggs in frittatas.
- Serve yoghurt and cheese as snacks.

- Add nuts to baked goods, salads and trail mixes. Check if your tween's school has a ban on nuts before packing their lunch box!
- Use legumes, such as chickpeas, red kidney beans or cannellini beans, in patties, rice salads or pasta salads.

Complex carbohydrates

Adequate carbohydrates, or carbs, are necessary to fuel busy bodies and brains and supply B vitamins, which are used by the body to convert food into energy. Carbs also supply fibre, which helps children maintain a healthy digestive system.

Example food sources: brown rice, quinoa, wholemeal pasta, brown rice noodles, legumes (also a protein), sweet potato, oats, wholegrain bread, wholegrain wraps, and fruit.

Using complex carbs in meals/snacks:

- Offer fruit as a snack.
- Make a mini Bircher muesli using oats and fruit for morning tea.
- Have wraps or sandwiches for lunch.
- Try brown rice, quinoa or pasta salads with roasted sweet potato.

Healthy fats

The brain is mostly made up of fat, so it makes sense that healthy fats are needed for brain function and development.

Example food sources: fatty fish (such as salmon or tuna), avocado, extra-virgin olive oil, nuts and seeds.

Using healthy fats in meals/snacks:

- Add salmon or tuna to wraps, sandwiches and salads, or mash them with avocado to spread on crackers.
- Use nuts and seeds in baked goods. If your tween's school bans nuts, just use seeds!
- Turn avocado into guacamole and serve it with crackers or vegetable sticks.
- Drizzle a bit of extra-virgin olive oil over salads and pasta dishes, or use it in dips such as hummus.

Calcium

Calcium is required for the normal development and maintenance of the skeleton, in addition to proper nervous and cardiac system function. During childhood and adolescence, adequate calcium is necessary to ensure peak bone mass density is achieved.

Example food sources: dairy (milk, cheese, yoghurt), canned salmon with bones, dried figs, broccoli, bok choy, tofu set with calcium, almonds, tahini and oats.

Using calcium in meals/snacks:

- Add baked tofu to salads, or simply eat it as a little snack.
- Add dried figs to trail mixes and baked goods.
- Serve cheese with crackers or vegetables as a snack.
- Add yoghurt or tahini to dips such as beetroot dip.

Iron

Iron is a mineral that is vital for transporting oxygen around the body, as well as red blood cells and energy production. If iron levels are low, it can result in feelings of fatigue and lethargy.

Example food sources: beef, lamb, sardines, canned salmon, chicken, lentils, tahini, dried apricots, almonds, spinach and wheatgerm.

Using iron in meals/snacks:

- Turn beef or lamb into mini meatballs.
- Use salmon in salads or dips, or turn it into patties.
- Use chicken in wraps, sandwiches and salads.
- Make hummus using tahini.
- Add spinach to wraps and salads.
- Add wheatgerm to bliss balls or baked goods.

Zinc

Zinc is a mineral, and a co-factor or 'helper molecule' for more than 300 enzymes and proteins involved in many important bodily functions, necessary for cell growth and immunity.

Example food sources: beef, capsicum, egg yolks, milk, sunflower and pumpkin seeds, whole grains and seafood.

Using zinc in meals/snacks:

- Make a frittata using roasted capsicum, milk and eggs and serve with a salad sprinkled with whole grains and seeds.
- Make a trail mix using sunflower and pumpkin seeds.
- Use nut flours in baked goods.
- Make a smoothie, adding dark cacao, yoghurt and your tween's favourite fruits.
- Make porridge with chia seeds, full-cream milk, hemp seeds and dates.

What about fussy eaters?

Children who are less than enthusiastic when it comes to mealtimes or very particular about the types of food they will or won't eat can cause much stress in the kitchen. Parents may be fearful that their fussy eater is not eating what they should, or as much as they should. Food preferences begin in infancy and carry through childhood into adulthood, making it all the more important to help your child develop healthy habits when it comes to food early on in life!

Getting to know your child's preferences, habits and behaviours around food is critical if you want them to enjoy a wide variety of foods. Keep a food diary: it will help you to understand your child's appetite and avoid unrealistic expectations at mealtimes. Play games with food to allow your child to experience food and develop their own taste preferences. Have conversations with your child about their likes and dislikes and encourage them to get creative and experiment with their own edible combinations. All of these ideas help with their sensory processing of food, which is believed to be a large contributor to eating preferences.

If you are at a loss with your fussy eater and seeking some inspiration, here are some easy ways to introduce more healthy foods into your child's diet:

- Stir ground-up flaxseeds into porridge or muesli.
- Blitz vegetables in a food processor and use the puree as a base for risotto.
- Make iceblocks from yoghurt blended with fruit.
- Opt for vegetable-based dips – roast beetroot, roast pumpkin or mashed avocado.
- Try a zucchini slice or frittata, with grated zucchini and carrot.
- Spread sandwiches with hummus, avocado or cannellini bean dip.
- Serve pasta with a nutrient-dense puree such as pumpkin and lentil.
- Make smoothies with milk, yoghurt, chia seeds, oats and fresh fruit.

Tweens 7-Day Sample Meal Plan

	Day 1	Day 2	Day 3	Day 4	Day 5	Day 6	Day 7
Breakfast	Berry & Beetroot Smoothie (p. 107) + optional piece of toast with avocado or cheese	Raw Fruit Breakfast Crumble (p. 119)	Golden Kiwi & Raspberry 'Cream' Oats (p. 132)	Golden Kiwi & Raspberry 'Cream' Oats (p. 132)	Vegan Apple & Cinnamon Nut Chia Oat Pudding (p. 139)	Raw Fruit Breakfast Crumble (p. 119)	Fresh Coconut & Chia Bowl (p. 120)
Snack (optional)	Avocado Edamame Hummus (p. 154) with veggie sticks and rice crackers	Piece of fruit with coconut yoghurt	Vegetable juice with beetroot, carrot and pink grapefruit	Seed crackers with avocado	Quick Carrot Hummus (p. 252) with veggie sticks and rice crackers	Piece of fruit with almonds	Berry & Beetroot Smoothie (p. 107)
Lunch	Rainbow Legume Pasta Salad (p. 184) + trail mix and/or popcorn	Leftover Rainbow Legume Pasta Salad + trail mix and/or popcorn	Quinoa, Herb, Pea & Ricotta Frittatas (p. 190) + homemade roasted sweet potato chips with hummus or salsa	Salad, egg and cheese wrap + trail mix and/or popcorn	Salad, egg and cheese wrap + trail mix and/or popcorn	Japanese Rice Cones (p. 246) + trail mix and/or popcorn	Chickpea & Quinoa Greek Salad (p. 165) + trail mix and/or popcorn
Snack (optional)	Carrot Mini Muffins with Cashew Icing (p. 280)	Leftover Carrot Mini Muffins with Cashew Icing	Immune Supportive Manuka Smoothie (p. 110)	Pear, Banana & Blueberry Muffins (p. 290)	Leftover Pear, Banana & Blueberry Muffins	Berry & Beetroot Smoothie (p. 107)	Seed crackers with cheese and tomato
Dinner	Baked Barramundi with Honey Carrots (p. 201) + steamed veggies and rice V: tofu	Spelt Gnocchi with Rich Tomato Sauce (p. 234) + steamed veggies	Spring Lamb Cottage Pie with Cauliflower Top (p. 232) + steamed veggies and corn V: lentils	Spaghetti with Mushroom & Tofu Balls (p. 222)	Cashew-Crumbed Salmon Lettuce Cups (p. 199) + steamed rice V: tofu	Smoked Paprika Fish Tacos with Tomato Salsa (p. 230) V: tofu or veggie patty	Coconut Chicken Nuggets (p. 208) + salad/ veggies and roasted potato V: tofu
Supper (optional)	Chocolate & Coconut-Dipped Frozen Fruit (p. 282)	Hot coconut milk with cinnamon and raw honey	Apple with nut butter	Berries with coconut yoghurt and crushed nuts	Milk with cacao and honey	Yoghurt and fruit	Berries with coconut yoghurt and crushed nuts

Case Study – Tween

Sophie is ten years old. She and her mother came to see me at my nutrition practice as her mother was concerned that Sophie was constantly tired and not sleeping well. Sophie is slightly above the healthy weight range for her height. She is a fussy eater and was only eating bland, starchy foods and some fruits with a high glycaemic content. She would often say she was feeling sick in the morning and didn't want to go to school, but she eventually confided in her mum that she was being bullied at school.

Nutrition

In our first session, I advised that Sophie go for a full blood test and get her zinc and magnesium levels checked out. Overall, her blood test results were within the normal range for her age, but, as suspected, her zinc and magnesium levels were low.

We started putting a program in place to address these mineral deficiencies and other health issues that Sophie was experiencing. Educating Sophie and her mum about the importance of balanced nutrition was vital. I explained the role of different nutrients, and together we explored other aspects of functional nutrition, such as learning about various food groups and concepts like the glycaemic index, identifying low- to moderate-GI foods, and how to read labels.

It was also important for Sophie and her family to start preparing meals together and sit down to eat with each other. Both the hands-on experience of making meals and eating together as a family help to foster positive connections to food. To make meals more interesting, I created a food plan for Sophie that gradually introduced new foods to her diet in simple and delicious ways yet was flexible enough to accommodate those times when she preferred more familiar ingredients.

We focused on foods that were high in the nutrients that Sophie was lacking: zinc and magnesium. Zinc deficiency can affect immune health as well as a person's sense of taste and smell, while a deficiency in magnesium can manifest as fatigue, metabolic irregularities and even symptoms of depression.

To supplement Sophie's diet, I added in a plant-based chocolate protein powder (packed with B vitamins and magnesium) and tasteless zinc drops to be mixed into a smoothie, which she has for breakfast and sometimes takes to school as a snack. Before bed each night, Sophie's mum makes her a warm almond milk drink, adding a little magnesium powder and cinnamon, which helps improve Sophie's sleep and anxiety.

Movement

Sophie and her mum started going for more walks outdoors together, which gave them the opportunity to chat and bond in the fresh air and sunshine. Sophie also joined the school netball team and has been enthusiastically participating in the games and training sessions, which is helping to improve her fitness.

Mind

Sophie's mum has been meditating with her on the weekends, using the meditation app Headspace. The app has meditations specifically targeted at kids, which Sophie enjoys and finds soothing. She has also started having sessions with her school counsellor, whom she says she really likes. The counsellor has been helping Sophie to recognise when she is feeling anxious and has given her some practical tools to cope with those feelings. The counsellor has also explained to Sophie that it is normal to feel uncomfortable at times.

Sophie has begun reciting a positive mantra whenever she feels lonely and practising 'box breathing' (see p. 18) when she feels anxious. She has also been listening to calming music at night, to wind down for bed. All these techniques have helped her to feel more at ease and in control, knowing that whenever anxiety stirs up, she has the tools to help herself calm down.

Mantra – Breathe in and out. Change is a fun adventure that you will conquer. I am my own best friend.

Connection

When Sophie joined the school netball team, not only did her fitness levels improve, but she also met several lovely girls who she feels are like her, and they have become firm friends. Being part of a supportive social group has increased Sophie's self-confidence and resilience, helping her become more assertive and stand up for herself, until the bullies no longer saw her as an easy target and began to back off. She now looks forward to going to school each morning.

Conventional Medicine

Sophie went for a follow-up blood test six months later, to recheck her zinc and magnesium levels, which happily are settling into the normal range for her age. I recommended that Sophie repeat these tests on an annual basis, to keep on top of her overall health.

Teenagers

Ah, the teenage years ... a time of roller-coaster emotions, raging hormones and self-discovery. Whether you're a late bloomer, like I was, or an early starter in the world of puberty, these years represent a significant chapter in a human's life journey.

As a teenager, I felt like my development was all over the place. I was flat-chested and got my period late, but I had a growth spurt early and was taller than most of my peers; I looked mature for my age but felt young internally. I frequently felt anxious and had difficulties going to sleep. And while I formed many beautiful friendships that remain solid to this day, I often felt like I didn't fit in. Fortunately, there was one place where I always felt like I belonged: the kitchen. I'd be in there every day after school, conjuring up tasty titbits from whatever wholefood ingredients I could find in the pantry and fridge. My hormones might have been unpredictable, but the daily ritual of cooking (and eating) nutritious homemade snacks brought me much comfort and pleasure – and although I didn't know it at the time, that ritual was setting the building blocks of a solid 'food foundation' and kept the puberty blues at bay.

Puberty, the remarkable period of transition from childhood to adulthood, opens up a world of new experiences and challenges. The journey is marked by several biological milestones, differentiated by gender.

	Female	*Male*
Puberty and reproductive readiness	As girls enter puberty, hormonal changes orchestrated by the brain's hypothalamus bring on the onset of the menstrual cycle. A monthly surge in LH and FSH triggers your ovaries to release an egg, and the subsequent rise and fall of oestrogen and progesterone prepare the lining of your womb for pregnancy. If the egg is not fertilised, the lining of the womb is shed when you have your period.	As boys enter puberty, the brain's hypothalamus triggers the release of LH and FSH, causing the testes to produce testosterone and oestrogen, setting the stage for the physical changes to come.
Visible changes	The signs of puberty are your body's way of letting you know that amazing changes are underway. From the start of your menstrual cycle to breast development, acne, growth spurts, body odour, pubic hair and even vaginal discharge – these are all natural parts of your body's growth.	The male journey includes a voice that deepens, an increase in body size, the development of pubic hair and the enlargement of the testes and scrotum. Increased oil production can sometimes lead to acne, another marker of this stage.

While the biological paths of female and male teenagers have distinctly different features, they do have something in common: regardless of sex, all teenage bodies are undergoing immense growth and development. The growth spurts and changes that you experience demand extra energy, protein, vitamins and minerals ... and as your intake needs increase, it is essential to nourish your body with the right nutrients.

While diet and healthy life choices are critical, sleep is also essential at this stage. Growth hormone, released during sleep, is crucial for bone and muscle development. It also aids in regulating hormones related to mood and stress, which is so important during the emotional and physical changes teenagers go through. During puberty there is a shift in the circadian rhythm, causing melatonin to be released later in the evening, which is why so many teenagers become night owls, so they might need a bit of extra sleep in the morning.

Remember, this is the time to prioritise healthy eating and sufficient sleep to optimise those hormones so critical to supporting your body's growth.

Hormone Supportive Foods

These foods are supportive for teenagers in terms of balancing hormones and overall health due to the various nutrients and compounds they contain:

- **Hemp Seeds:** Hemp seeds are rich in omega-3 and omega-6 fatty acids, which are essential for hormone production and regulation. They also provide plant-based protein and minerals that support overall growth and development.
- **Nuts:** Nuts, such as almonds and walnuts, are packed with healthy fats, vitamins and minerals. They provide essential nutrients for hormone synthesis and are a convenient snack for sustaining energy levels throughout the day.
- **Avocado:** Avocado is a great source of healthy fats, particularly monounsaturated fats, which are important for hormone production and maintaining overall health. It also provides vitamins and minerals that support skin health and growth.
- **Salmon and Tuna:** Fatty fish like salmon and tuna are excellent sources of omega-3 fatty acids, which play a role in regulating hormones and reducing inflammation. These fish also provide high-quality protein necessary for growth and repair.
- **Chicken:** Lean poultry like chicken is a good source of protein, which is essential for muscle development and overall growth. It also contains important B vitamins that support energy metabolism.
- **Whole Grains:** Whole grains like brown rice, quinoa, buckwheat and oats provide complex carbohydrates and fibre. These foods help maintain stable blood sugar levels, which can positively impact hormonal balance and energy throughout the day.
- **Leafy Greens:** Leafy greens like spinach and kale are rich in vitamins, minerals and antioxidants. These nutrients support overall health and can help with hormone regulation.
- **Legumes and pulses:** Legumes, including beans and lentils, are excellent sources of plant-based protein, fibre and various vitamins and minerals. They contribute to balanced energy levels and support overall growth.
- **Red Meat:** Red meat, such as lean beef, is a valuable source of iron, zinc and protein. Iron is particularly important for teenagers, especially girls, to prevent anaemia and support growth.

- **Seafood:** Seafood, besides being a source of omega-3 fatty acids, provides minerals like iodine, which is crucial for thyroid hormone production and regulation.
- **Pumpkin Seeds:** Pumpkin seeds are rich in zinc, a mineral that plays a role in hormone production and immune function. They are also a good source of healthy fats and protein.
- **Chia Seeds:** Chia seeds are high in omega-3 fatty acids, fibre and antioxidants. They support digestion and provide essential nutrients for hormonal balance.
- **Natural Yoghurt:** Natural yoghurt contains probiotics that promote gut health. A healthy gut microbiome can indirectly influence hormonal balance and overall wellbeing.
- **Kefir:** Kefir is a probiotic-rich fermented milk drink that supports gut health and may have a positive impact on hormonal regulation.
- **Vegetables and Fruits:** Vegetables and fruits of all kinds are rich in vitamins, minerals, antioxidants and fibre. They contribute to overall health and can help maintain stable blood sugar levels.

Including a variety of these foods in a balanced diet can provide the necessary nutrients and support hormonal balance during the crucial teenage years when growth and development are at their peak. It's important for teenagers to maintain a well-rounded diet to support their overall health and wellbeing.

Teens 7-Day Sample Meal Plan

	Day 1	Day 2	Day 3	Day 4	Day 5	Day 6	Day 7
Breakfast	Golden Kiwi and Raspberry 'Cream' Oats (p. 132)	Lemon & Coconut Buckwheat Porridge (p. 118)	Eggs on seeded toast with avocado	Eggs on seeded toast with avocado	Lemon & Coconut Buckwheat Porridge (p. 118)	Healthy Chocolate Protein Pancakes (p. 126)	Fresh Coconut & Chia Bowl (p. 120)
Snack (optional)	Avocado Edamame Hummus (p. 154) with veggie sticks and rice crackers + yoghurt	Leftover Avocado Edamame Hummus with veggie sticks and rice crackers + yoghurt	Cheese and tomato on wholegrain crackers + a piece of fruit	Cheese and tomato on wholegrain crackers + a piece of fruit	Quick Carrot Hummus (p. 252) with veggie sticks and rice crackers + a piece of fruit	Apple with nut butter and popcorn	Apple with nut butter and popcorn
Lunch	Leek, Macadamia & Turmeric Frittatas (p. 170) + buckwheat pasta tossed with pesto and cherry tomatoes	Leftover Leek, Macadamia & Turmeric Frittatas + buckwheat pasta tossed with pesto and cherry tomatoes	Salad and avocado wrap with your protein of choice + trail mix	Salad and avocado wrap with your protein of choice + trail mix	Chickpea & Quinoa Greek Salad (p. 165) + popcorn	Super Sausage & Mushroom Rolls (p. 192) + salad and a piece of fruit	Egg Nutty Lunch Bowl with Creamy Avocado Dressing (p. 156) + trail mix
Snack (optional)	Banana Chocolate Muffins with Maple Cream Cheese Frosting (p. 273) + a piece of fruit	Leftover Banana Chocolate Muffins with Maple Cream Cheese Frosting + a piece of fruit	Brain-Boosting Smoothie (p. 107)	Acai & Berry Smoothie Bowl with Acai Choc Crumble (p. 117)	Acai & Berry Smoothie Bowl with Acai Choc Crumble (p. 117)	Quick Carrot Hummus (p. 252) with veggie sticks and rice crackers + yoghurt	Yoghurt with fruit with nut/seed sprinkle and granola
Dinner	Cashew-Crumbed Salmon Lettuce Cups (p. 199) V: tofu	Chia Beef Burger with Apple & Beetroot Relish (p. 162) + a side salad and roasted sweet potato fries	Spring Lamb Cottage Pie with Cauliflower Top (p. 232) + steamed veggies V: lentils	Smoked Paprika Fish Tacos with Tomato Salsa (p. 230) V: mushrooms	Mini Spicy Chicken, Beetroot & Goat's Cheese Pizza (p. 214) + a side salad V: tofu	Chicken Thighs with Mushroom Sauce (p. 226) + steamed veggies V: chickpeas	Chickpea, Tofu & Spinach Pasta (p. 235)
Supper (optional)	Yoghurt and fruit + popcorn	Chocolate & Coconut-Dipped Frozen Fruit (p. 282)	Apple with nut butter	Yoghurt and berries	Lemon Hemp Bliss Balls (p. 287)	Homemade Chocolate Nut Coconut Bars (p. 285)	Leftover Lemon Hemp Bliss Balls

Case Study – Teen

Kate is a 13-year-old girl who recently started Year 7. When she came to see me, she had been diagnosed with anaemia and was struggling with sleep. She had also been coping with the discomfort of painful periods since she began menstruating a year ago.

Kate hadn't been eating a balanced diet, and she had stopped eating red meat, which exacerbated the situation. This was likely contributing to her lack of energy, feelings of fatigue and low mood. Her difficulty sleeping could have been due to various factors, including stress, hormonal changes and discomfort from her menstrual pain. Kate's severe menstrual pain affected her quality of life and sometimes led to missed schooldays and reduced participation in daily activities.

Nutrition

In my consulting sessions with Kate, I focused on the basics of nutrition: understanding food groups, labels on food packaging and the glycaemic index. I also advised Kate that all meals must have balanced amounts of lean protein, good fats and low-GI carbohydrates.

To address her anaemia, I developed a food plan rich in iron and vitamin B12: lean meats, beans, leafy greens, nuts, seeds and fortified cereals. We concentrated on getting her eating regularly to help sustain her energy levels, and cut out most processed foods – although Kate still indulges in chocolate occasionally, she now has dark chocolate and combines it with a small handful of fruit or nuts. As another simple 'energy-levelling' swap, she drinks green tea with raw honey instead of coffee with sugar.

We also introduced supplements to her diet: iron, to target her anaemia, as well as magnesium and vitex, a herb, to help alleviate her painful periods.

Movement

Kate has joined her school rowing team and is loving the regular physical activity, which is improving her strength and energy levels; she also loves the team spirit, which is helping her feel more included socially. When Kate has her period, she now opts for gentle exercise like yoga or walking, as she finds it helps reduce her menstrual pain.

Mind

Kate has been exploring mindfulness practices like meditation using the app Insight Timer. She has started meditating while on the bus to school in the mornings, which she says chills her out before class.

She has also benefited from learning stress-management techniques and putting them into practice: journalling, 'triangle breathing' (see p. 18) and avoiding her devices and screens for at least 90 minutes before bedtime most nights – all which have enhanced her sleep quality and overall mood.

Mantra – Celebrate and revel in your uniqueness.

Connection

Since Kate joined her school rowing team, she has loved the camaraderie of the group and made new friends. She has also joined the school drama club, which has helped her increase her confidence and learn to express herself.

Conventional Medicine

Kate goes for regular blood tests now, every three to six months, to monitor her iron levels.

Overall, Kate's iron levels have improved, as have her energy levels. Her menstrual cycle is less painful and irregular. She feels more knowledgeable about what to eat, as well as when and how to cope with stress to help her body.

Adult Women, 18–40

My personal journey to motherhood was a rocky one: finding out at 29 years old that I couldn't have children naturally was a mind explosion. There was a lot of shame, anger, confusion and overall sadness. Six rounds of in-vitro fertilisation (IVF) treatments and three miscarriages later, my husband and I eventually had our amazing daughter. In total, the whole process took us five years. As a practising nutritionist, my focus had always been on how to best support my clients through their weight-loss journey, but I wish I had known more back then about the way stress hormones impact reproduction and our ability to have offspring.

For women, the years between 18 and 40 are a dynamic stage of life, filled with physical, emotional and lifestyle changes. For maximum wellbeing, you need to think holistically. There are many different kinds of health, all of them important:

Physical and preventive health: You need to eat a balanced diet, stay hydrated, engage in regular physical activity and get quality sleep. Regular check-ups and screenings are important, and this is also a crucial time to build and maintain strong bones. Make weight-bearing exercises a part of your regular workouts, and don't forget to get enough calcium and vitamin D!

Mental and emotional health: Whether you're studying or working, starting a family or bringing up kids, stress, anxiety or depression can be part of the package. Seeking support, practising stress-management techniques and finding that perfect work-life balance are vital, and you should never underestimate the power of a supportive social circle!

Society's beauty standards can also place a lot of pressure on you, so always remember that you are beautiful as you are. A positive self-image and self-care should always be high on the list.

Sexual and reproductive health: Keeping track of your menstrual cycle, managing PMS symptoms and dealing with menstrual pain are also part of the package in your reproductive years, as are contraception and family planning. Even if fertility isn't your primary concern, safe sex and effective contraception are important. Regular screenings and awareness about sexually transmitted infections (STIs) also contribute to your sexual health.

Sleep: In all stages, just like a healthy diet and regular physical activity, sleep is critical for a healthy body and mind. Getting enough sleep helps support the production and regulation of hormones like cortisol, which influences stress response, and growth hormone, which impacts overall health. Waking up not feeling refreshed and feeling exhausted throughout the day can leave you feeling blah and may disrupt hormonal balance, impact mood, food choice, overall productivity and reproductive hormones.

The key, as always, is to prioritise self-care, listen to your body and seek medical advice when needed. Remember that everyone's journey is unique – this is your time, so make the most of it and give yourself support when needed.

The Fertile Years

The decision to become a parent is a profound one, but it's just the start of a long journey: first there's the delicate dance of fertility and conception, then, if all goes to plan, pregnancy and, eventually, the miraculous event of childbirth. These days many women juggle paid work with family planning, adding a huge amount of pressure to both, but we also have more control over our fertility than ever before. In this section, we'll look at the pivotal role hormones play in this journey, and explore some of the new options available to women now, such as freezing eggs for later use.

A hormonal balancing act

Women are at their most fertile between their late teens and early 30s. Achieving a healthy balance of three primary sex hormones – oestrogen, progesterone and testosterone – is fundamental to fertility and a successful pregnancy. Unfortunately, the modern lifestyle can be laden with stress, lack of sleep, poor diet and exposure to pollution or hormone-disrupting chemicals such as xenoestrogens, which can throw out this finely calibrated hormonal equilibrium.

Some signs of low oestrogen are:

- hot flushes
- sleep disturbances
- dry skin
- foggy thinking
- heart palpitations

- painful intercourse
- night sweats
- vaginal dryness/atrophy
- headaches
- memory lapses
- yeast infections
- low mood.

Some signs of elevated oestrogen or 'oestrogen dominance' are:

- water retention
- breast swelling and tenderness
- heavy, irregular periods
- fatigue
- sugar cravings
- weight gain
- fibrocystic breasts
- mood swings
- uterine fibroids
- low thyroid levels
- nervousness/anxiety/irritability
- facial flushing.

Stress and hormonal health

One major player that often disrupts hormonal harmony is cortisol – the body's primary stress hormone. Excessive cortisol production due to chronic stress can lead to a cascade of hormonal imbalances. Of particular concern is its impact on progesterone production. Progesterone is essential for preparing and maintaining the uterine lining for a fertilised egg. When cortisol steals the spotlight, progesterone production can take a hit, leading to anovulation – a condition in which ovulation doesn't occur, impacting fertility. Techniques for managing stress, such as mindfulness, yoga and meditation, can help regulate cortisol levels and protect progesterone production.

The Modern Choice: Freezing Eggs

In recent years, advancements in medical technology have introduced a new potential step in a woman's reproductive journey – the option to freeze eggs. This practice involves retrieving a woman's eggs, freezing them and storing them for future use. Egg freezing offers women the chance to preserve their fertility, allowing them to pursue their education, career or personal goals without the pressure of age-related fertility decline. By freezing eggs during their prime reproductive years, women can put off starting a family until they're ready, even if that time comes after their natural fertility has decreased.

Setting the stage for a smooth transition

Supporting women hormonally during their reproductive years has benefits that go on far beyond conception and pregnancy, helping to pave the way for a smoother experience of perimenopause and menopause – the stages that follow the fertile years.

The Menstrual Cycle

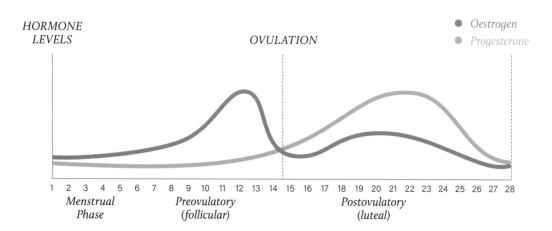

The graph shows the rise and fall of oestrogen and progesterone over the course of a woman's menstrual cycle. Not all menstrual cycles look or feel the same, but they typically follow the same hormonal rhythm.

This graph shows an average 28-day cycle, including the:

Menstrual phase: The menstrual phase, aka the period, starts on the first day of bleeding and ends when the bleeding stops. This is when oestrogen and progesterone levels are at their lowest.

Preovulatory phase: Also known as the follicular phase, the preovulatory phase also starts on the first day of the period and ends with ovulation. During this time, follicle-stimulating hormone (FSH) is released to make the eggs inside the ovaries develop, and the uterus lining thickens. Oestrogen levels rise during this phase.

Ovulation: During ovulation, a surge of luteinising hormone (LH) triggers the release of a mature egg from an ovary towards the uterus. Oestrogen levels decline post ovulation.

Postovulatory phase: Also known as the luteal phase, the postovulatory phase lasts until the beginning of the next period. This is when progesterone levels rise to support the thickening of the uterus lining and prepare for a fertilised egg to implant. If fertilisation does not occur, the uterus lining is shed and the cycle begins again.

Hormone Supportive Foods

These foods are excellent choices for supporting hormonal health in adult women aged 18 to 40, because they provide essential nutrients and health-promoting compounds that are particularly beneficial during the various stages of their menstrual cycle:

- **Avocado:** Avocado is a source of monounsaturated fats that support hormone production and overall health. Healthy fats are crucial for the synthesis of hormones.
- **Fatty Fish (Salmon):** Fatty fish like salmon provide omega-3 fatty acids, which help regulate hormones and reduce inflammation. Omega-3s are important for menstrual cycle regularity and overall hormonal balance.
- **Nuts/Seeds:** Nuts and seeds offer healthy fats, vitamins, minerals and fibre. They provide essential nutrients for hormone synthesis and are convenient snacks for sustaining energy levels.
- **Extra-Virgin Olive Oil (EVOO):** EVOO contains monounsaturated fats and antioxidants that support hormone balance and reduce inflammation. It's a key component of the Mediterranean diet, which is known for its hormone-supporting properties.

- **Fruits and Vegetables:** A diet rich in a variety of fruits and vegetables provides essential vitamins, minerals, antioxidants and fibre. These nutrients support overall health and hormone regulation and help manage menstrual symptoms.
- **Cocoa/Cacao:** Cocoa and cacao contain compounds that can have mood-improving effects and provide a tasty option for those cravings during the menstrual cycle.
- **Whole Grains:** Whole grains, like brown rice and oats, offer complex carbohydrates and fibre, which can help stabilise blood sugar levels. This is important for hormonal balance and maintaining steady energy.
- **Lean Protein:** Lean sources of protein such as fish, chicken, eggs and natural yoghurt provide essential amino acids necessary for hormone synthesis and muscle repair.
- **Fermented Foods:** Fermented foods like kefir, sauerkraut, kimchi and kombucha support gut health, which can indirectly influence hormonal balance and overall wellbeing.
- **Herbs and Spices:** Many herbs and spices have health-promoting properties and can be used to flavour dishes without adding extra calories. They can enhance the taste of meals while providing potential health benefits.

Including these foods in a balanced diet can help adult women in their reproductive years maintain healthy hormonal balance, support regular menstrual cycles and promote overall wellbeing. Remember that individual dietary needs and preferences may vary, so it is important to consult a healthcare provider, registered nutritionist or dietitian for personalised guidance on optimising hormonal health.

Female Adults (General) 7-Day Sample Meal Plan

	Day 1	Day 2	Day 3	Day 4	Day 5	Day 6	Day 7
Upon waking	Lemon juice or apple cider vinegar in warm water	Lemon juice or apple cider vinegar in warm water	Lemon juice or apple cider vinegar in warm water	Lemon juice or apple cider vinegar in warm water	Lemon juice or apple cider vinegar in warm water	Lemon juice or apple cider vinegar in warm water	Lemon juice or apple cider vinegar in warm water
Breakfast	Healthy Chocolate Protein Pancakes (p. 126)	Lemon & Coconut Buckwheat Porridge (p. 118)	Lemon & Coconut Buckwheat Porridge (p. 118)	Immune Supportive Manuka Smoothie (p. 110)	Fresh Coconut & Chia Bowl (p. 120)	Buckwheat & Maca Crepes with Honey Whipped Ricotta & Roasted Berries (p. 277)	Miso Mushroom Scrambled Eggs (p. 142) + optional seeded toast
Snack (optional)	Piece of fruit and unsweetened yoghurt	Piece of fruit and unsweetened yoghurt	Leftover **Macadamia Nut Pâté** with veggie sticks	Roasted Beetroot & Hemp Seed Hummus (p. 250) on corn thins with avocado	Leftover Roasted Beetroot & Hemp Seed Hummus on corn thins with avocado	Leftover **Pear, Banana & Blueberry Muffins**	Unsweetened yoghurt with berries and nuts/seeds
Lunch	Egg Nutty Lunch Bowl with Creamy Avocado Dressing (p. 156)	Aromatic Indian Spinach & Coconut Soup (p. 152)	Leftover Aromatic Indian Spinach & Coconut Soup	Warm Charred Broccoli Salad with Herb Dressing (p. 159)	Salad and avocado wrap with your protein of choice	Salad and avocado wrap with your protein of choice	Broccolini, Brazil Nut & Quinoa Salad with Crispy Halloumi (p. 158) V: tofu
Snack (optional)	Macadamia Nut Pâté (p. 254) with veggie sticks	Leftover Macadamia Nut Pâté with veggie sticks	Piece of fruit and unsweetened yoghurt	Piece of fruit and unsweetened yoghurt	Pear, Banana & Blueberry Muffins (p. 290)	Piece of fruit and unsweetened yoghurt	Leftover **Pear, Banana & Blueberry Muffins**
Dinner	Sumac Lamb Fillets with Cauliflower Tabouli & Coconut Tzatziki (p. 233) V: veggie patty	Warm Ginger Satay Chicken Salad with Turmeric Cauliflower (p. 206) V: tofu	Cashew-Crumbed Salmon Lettuce Cups (p. 199) + optional steamed rice V: mushrooms	Quick Tomato, Walnut & Chickpea Stew (p. 218) + leafy salad and optional quinoa	Smoked Paprika Fish Tacos with Tomato Salsa (p. 230) V: tofu	Green Curry with Tofu, Peas & Capsicum (p. 212)	Warm Salmon & Zucchini Noodle Salad with Spicy Cashew Dressing (p. 205) V: tofu
Supper (optional)	Herbal tea and 2 squares of dark chocolate	Unsweetened yoghurt with berries and nuts/seeds	Cacao Beet Brownies (p. 279)	Unsweetened yoghurt with berries and nuts/seeds	Herbal tea and 2 squares of dark chocolate	Unsweetened yoghurt with berries and nuts/seeds	Leftover Cacao Beet Brownies

Case Study – Young Female Adult

Gina is a 22-year-old female who is studying full-time and working part-time. She is a high achiever but struggles with fatigue, mild heart palpitations, anxiety and depression. She finds it hard to self-regulate when stressed and is more prone to constipation. Her sleeping patterns are irregular, as she often gets home late from work or study and finds it difficult to wind down for bed. She has PCOS (polycystic ovary syndrome) and has been on the oral contraceptive pill since she was 16, primarily to help regulate her periods and reduce pain. She has healthy relationships with her family and boyfriend. Her aim is to lose weight, increase her self-confidence and establish a successful diet to help her meet her daily study and work demands.

On my advice, Gina scheduled an appointment with her GP to assess her insulin resistance, hormone levels and overall health. The results showed her overall health was good, but her fasting insulin level was high, indicating possible insulin resistance. Her ferritin levels were low, suggesting possible anaemia.

Creating a healthy plan for a young female adult with insulin resistance, irregular periods, high stress and weight gain involves a holistic approach that addresses various aspects of her lifestyle. Educating Gina about her digestion and menstrual cycle and what foods help support these processes has also helped relieve her constipation.

Note: Every woman's experience is different, but generally speaking women can experience changes in bowel habits over the menstrual cycle, because oestrogen and progesterone can inhibit smooth muscle contraction and therefore gastrointestinal motility.

It has been reported that significantly longer gut transit time occurs during the luteal phase than the follicular phase, which may lead to constipation.

Conversely, during the lead-up to and during menstruation, women may experience diarrhoea and/or loose stools. This is due to a drop in progesterone and also increased release of prostaglandins. Specifically, prostaglandins are released to cause the muscles of the uterus to contract and shed its lining. Prostaglandins affect the muscles of the gut, and diarrhoea is caused by increased muscle contractions.

Nutrition

Weight management is crucial for improving insulin sensitivity and regulating hormones.

I mapped out a food plan for Gina that included the following:

- increased intake of vegetables, fruits, whole grains, lean proteins and healthy fats
- reduced intake of gluten, dairy, processed foods, sugary beverages, excessive added sugars, alcohol and caffeine, all of which can exacerbate stress and hormonal fluctuations
- swapping foods that are high on the glycaemic index with lower GI alternatives (e.g. switching from jasmine rice to quinoa and brown rice), to better manage insulin levels
- combining iron-rich foods with foods high in vitamin C, to aid iron absorption
- a focus on liver-supporting foods to assist in the detoxification process, such as legumes, which are a rich source of sulphur, unprocessed grains, good fats, citrus, and bitter lettuces such as rocket and chicory, to name just a few.

We also introduced some supplements to her diet:

- chromium, an essential mineral that works with insulin to help the body regulate blood sugar levels
- a vitamin B complex with a strong focus on B5 and B6 vitamins, to help with her stress and energy levels
- highly absorbable iron and vitamin C
- magnesium to give relief from cramping and stress and boost sleep.

Movement

Gina started funk dance classes twice a week and also began jogging, strength training and going on regular walks with her friends. Not only has the physical exercise improved her insulin sensitivity and aided in weight loss, the variety of activities that Gina is participating in and the opportunity they give her to socialise means that she is more likely to keep up her interests and efforts.

Mind

Gina has incorporated the stress-reducing practices of deep breathing exercises and mindfulness into her daily routine. She starts her mornings off by doing alternate nostril breathing (see p. 19), writing in her journal and reciting positive mantras. She has also been concentrating on building better sleep hygiene habits: no caffeine past 12 pm during the day, and turning the lights down early and playing relaxing music in the evenings, turning screens off by 9.30 pm and tucking herself in bed by 10.30 pm – all which have enhanced both her sleep quality and quantity.

Mantra – With knowledge comes power and an opportunity to create change.

Connection

Gina joined a five-day transcendental meditation workshop; this meditation technique involves silently repeating a specific mantra or sound to achieve a state of deep relaxation and inner peace. Gina also joined an online forum for people who were going through stressful situations. She loves the group forum, the daily quotes and mantras and feels like she has found like-minded women.

Conventional Medicine

Gina is still seeing her GP for regular six-monthly blood tests and check-ups. Staying up to date with regular health screenings to monitor her overall health allows her to address any potential issues promptly. On the recommendation of her GP, she also downloaded a period tracker, to help her keep track of her menstrual cycle, so she knows when she is due for her period or ovulating.

Overall, Gina is feeling confident about the changes she has made to her diet, and the exercise and lifestyle changes, although they took time to implement, have now become an easy routine. Her energy levels have remained mostly consistent; if they fall, or when she is stressed, she feels she now has the tools to support herself. After addressing her insulin resistance, the pain from the PCOS has improved.

Perimenopause

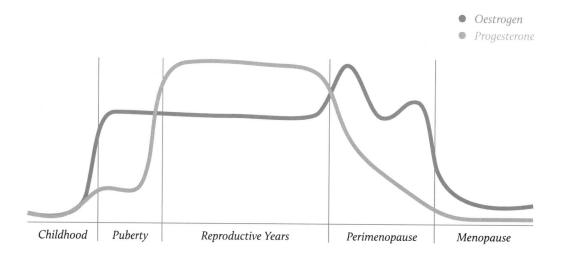

Oestrogen
Progesterone

| Childhood | Puberty | Reproductive Years | Perimenopause | Menopause |

This graph illustrates the natural rhythm of the two key reproductive hormones, oestrogen and progesterone, through the lifespan of a woman. As you read further into this book, you will learn how the rise and fall of these hormones play a role in perimenopause and menopause, and contribute to the various symptoms experienced by women during this change.

Several years ago, I was told by my doctor that I was going through perimenopause, which is the phase before menopause, typically occurring in the late 30s or early 40s. It involves hormonal fluctuations leading to irregular periods, mood swings and symptoms such as hot flushes.

It came as a surprise. Like so many other women my age, I was at the peak of my career, juggling work with caring for my young daughter and supporting my mother who was chronically unwell – all while desperately trying not to burn out. To add to the pressure, having another child was really important to my husband and me, and I was about to commence IVF treatment. It would have been my first round of IVF since giving birth to my daughter two years prior, but I had already gone through six cycles of IVF before then in my attempts to have children.

Being 39 years old at the time, I was shocked to be told that I was very unlikely to fall pregnant again. I thought I was too young to be perimenopausal. Perimenopause is a crucial – and often overlooked – phase in a woman's life that serves as a transition towards menopause, marking the gradual decline of reproductive hormones. This phase, which typically begins in a woman's 40s but can occur earlier or later, encompasses various physiological changes, primarily resulting from fluctuations in sex hormones, particularly oestrogen and progesterone.

Perimenopause often gets painted with a gloomy brush, focusing on the symptoms and hurdles it brings. But it's not all doom and gloom! In fact, for many women, perimenopause can be a time of positivity and empowerment. Age brings wisdom, and with it comes a boost in self-assurance. You start feeling more sure of yourself, thanks to the life experiences you've racked up. While you might struggle with mood swings, you may feel more comfortable expressing your feelings, leading to more open and honest communication with loved ones.

I didn't end up going through with that seventh IVF cycle in the end. After much self-reflection and many lengthy open, honest discussions with my husband, we decided that it was time to stop trying for more offspring. We realised how lucky we were to have what we already had, our beautiful little girl whom we adored and were utterly besotted with, and she was enough.

Perimenopause encourages you to become your own health champion, too. For example, sleep plays an important role, as the hormonal fluctuations you're experiencing , particularly oestrogen and progesterone, can disrupt sleep during this stage. Quality sleep becomes crucial for managing symptoms like hot flashes and mood swings, supporting your wellbeing.

Regular check-ups and screenings also become a priority, and there's a sense of satisfaction in taking control of your wellbeing. Perimenopause might just be the time when you and your body become the best of friends. You start to understand your needs and priorities better and get in touch with your body in a whole new way. It's like a personal journey of self-discovery, albeit sometimes a little overwhelming. Knowing that their hormones are up to some mischief, many women take the bull by the horns and prioritise self-care, including adopting healthier habits, hitting the gym and eating better. By shining a light on the positives and breaking through the fear and stigma, we can have more supportive and informed conversations about this natural phase in a woman's life.

Hormonal changes during perimenopause

If you're going through perimenopause, you'll know that it comes with a lot of physical and emotional changes. These changes are caused by a gradual decrease in the levels of certain sex hormones, which plays a pivotal role in driving the physiological shifts and symptoms you might be experiencing. These hormones include:

- **Oestrogen:** Oestrogen is a group of hormones, including oestradiol, oestrone and oestriol, primarily produced by the ovaries. In adult women, it plays a vital role in regulating the menstrual cycle, supporting bone health, maintaining the integrity of vaginal tissue and influencing mood and cognitive function. As women approach perimenopause, there is a decline in oestrogen production. Declining oestrogen levels are linked to symptoms such as irregular menstrual cycles, hot flushes, vaginal dryness, mood swings and more.

- **Progesterone:** Progesterone is another hormone produced by the ovaries, particularly during the second half of the menstrual cycle in preparation for a potential pregnancy. It helps regulate the uterine lining and supports pregnancy. In perimenopause, declining progesterone levels contribute to irregular menstrual cycles and mood changes, and may exacerbate symptoms like breast tenderness.

- **Testosterone:** While often associated with males, testosterone is also present in females, albeit in smaller amounts. It plays a role in maintaining libido, energy levels and overall wellbeing. During perimenopause, there can be a decline in testosterone production, which might contribute to low libido and reduced vitality.

- **Follicle-Stimulating Hormone (FSH) and Luteinising Hormone (LH):** FSH and LH are pituitary hormones that play a key role in regulating the menstrual cycle, stimulating the ovaries to produce oestrogen and progesterone. As the ovaries become less responsive to these hormones during perimenopause, their levels can fluctuate significantly, leading to irregular menstrual cycles and other symptoms.

- **Gonadotropin-Releasing Hormone (GnRH):** GnRH is a hormone released by the hypothalamus that triggers the release of FSH and LH from the pituitary gland. During perimenopause, the feedback loop between the ovaries, hypothalamus and pituitary gland becomes disrupted, leading to fluctuating levels of GnRH and subsequently impacting the regulation of other reproductive hormones.

Perimenopausal symptoms

Collectively, these fluctuating hormones contribute to the wide array of symptoms experienced during perimenopause. The symptoms can vary significantly from person to person, emphasising the need for a personalised approach to symptom management and support during this transformative period.

Some of the common symptoms include:

- **Irregular menstrual cycles:** Changes in hormone levels can lead to erratic menstrual cycles, with periods becoming shorter, longer, lighter or heavier.
- **Mood swings and irritability:** Hormonal imbalances can contribute to mood swings, irritability and increased emotional sensitivity.
- **Anxiety and depression:** Some women may experience heightened anxiety or even symptoms of depression due to hormonal fluctuations affecting neurotransmitter levels.
- **Hot flushes and night sweats:** These sudden episodes of intense heat, often followed by profuse sweating, are attributed to hormonal changes affecting the body's thermoregulation.
- **Sleep disturbances:** Hormonal fluctuations, particularly oestrogen and progesterone, can disrupt sleep during perimenopause. Changes during perimenopause can affect melatonin (sleep–wake hormone) production, potentially leading to difficulties falling asleep and staying asleep, as well as an increase in cortisol making it harder to sleep.
- **Weight gain:** Shifting hormones can contribute to weight gain, especially around the abdominal area.
- **Breast tenderness:** Hormonal fluctuations can lead to breast tenderness and discomfort.
- **Trouble concentrating:** Some women may experience difficulties with focus and concentration, often referred to as 'brain fog'.
- **Low libido:** Hormonal changes can contribute to a decreased interest in sexual activity.
- **Vaginal dryness:** Reduced oestrogen levels can lead to vaginal dryness and thinning of vaginal tissue, resulting in painful intercourse.
- **Urinary incontinence:** Changes in pelvic floor muscles and vaginal tissues can lead to bladder-control issues.
- **Joint pain:** Oestrogen aids in the production of lubricating fluid and reduces inflammation, so decreasing oestrogen levels can result in pain in the joints.

Diagnosis

Your GP or medical specialist can order blood tests to check your hormone levels. The tests they ask for will depend on the hormonal stage you are in and the symptoms you are experiencing. The most common baseline blood tests requested for perimenopause are outlined in the table below.

Perimenopause	*Thyroid Function*	*Cortisol*
Luteinising hormone (LH)	TSH	DHEAS
Follicle stimulating hormone (FSH)	Free T4	Cortisol
Oestradiol (E2)	Free T3	ACTH
Progesterone	Reverse T3	
Sex hormone–binding globulin (SHBG)	Thyroid antibodies (TPO Abs and Tg Abs)	
	Zinc	
	Iodine	
	Selenium	
	Iron	

There are also functional tests available that will give you a further picture of your hormonal health, including urinary cortisol, urinary iodine, urinary hormone and saliva testing for cortisol and sex hormones.

Managing perimenopausal symptoms

While perimenopause can be challenging, there are various strategies that women can adopt to alleviate symptoms and support their overall wellbeing:

- **Healthy diet:** A balanced diet rich in whole foods, lean proteins, healthy fats and a variety of nutrients can help support hormonal balance. Your liver is under more stress during perimenopause due to hormone fluctuation, and it needs support as it plays a crucial role in hormone metabolism, processing and clearing hormones from the bloodstream. Try nutrient-rich foods that contain antioxidants, anti-inflammatory properties and fibre, such as pineapple, lemons, grapefruit, pears, grapes, artichokes, shiitake mushrooms, garlic, carrot, beetroot, cucumber and bitter lettuces such as rocket and chicory. See below for more on eating to alleviate the symptoms of perimenopause.

- **Regular exercise:** Engaging in regular physical activity can help manage weight, improve mood and support overall hormonal health. Look at where you are in your life and choose the exercise which will best support that phase. For example, I now do more yoga, resistance training and short hill runs. This helps to keep me fit but doesn't overstimulate my adrenal glands like high-intensity cardiovascular exercise does.

- **Stress reduction:** Practices such as mindfulness, meditation and yoga can help reduce stress levels, which in turn can positively influence hormonal fluctuations.
- **Weight control:** Weight gained during perimenopause can exacerbate hormonal imbalances and worsen symptoms. Making changes to your diet and exercising regularly may help you to limit weight gain or maintain your current weight.
- **Supplements:** Some women may find relief from certain symptoms through supplements such as vitamin D, calcium and omega-3 fatty acids, as well as adding herbs such as black cohosh and sage, and adaptogenic herbs.
- **Plant-based solutions:** Herbal remedies like black cohosh and evening primrose oil have been explored for their potential to alleviate some perimenopausal symptoms.
- **Hormone replacement therapy (HRT):** In some cases, women may choose hormone replacement therapy to manage severe symptoms, taking prescribed hormones to supplement declining levels.

Overall, perimenopause is an amazing, transformative phase that deserves positive attention and understanding. It doesn't have to be spoken about in hushed tones – let's be loud and proud and acknowledge the hormonal shifts we are going through, together.

Eating to alleviate the symptoms of perimenopause

Eating a healthy, balanced diet is the best way to support your health as you go through perimenopause, but what you eat and when you eat can also help to alleviate perimenopausal symptoms.

Phytoestrogens: For some women, eating more foods containing phytoestrogens is helpful. Phytoestrogens are compounds found in plant and plant-derived foods that have a similar chemical structure to natural oestrogen and interact with oestrogen receptors in the body, mimicking the effect of natural oestrogen. Examples of foods rich in phytoestrogens include whole grains, soy products, flaxseeds, sesame seeds, chickpeas, lentils and other legumes, and certain fruits and vegetables. It's important to note, though, that some women may be sensitive to phytoestrogens and experience adverse effects. It's best to consult a healthcare provider or nutritionist for personalised advice before making any changes to your diet: you may need to limit your intake of certain phytoestrogens rather than increasing your intake.

Rethinking fasting: Intermittent fasting may have cardiometabolic and weight control benefits, but it can also be an added stress on the body. Some women can continue intermittent fasting during perimenopause without any negative effects, but those sensitive to stress and already experiencing poor sleep, fatigue and mood swings may find that fasting aggravates their symptoms. Fasting can, in some cases, further disrupt your hormonal balance and even put the thyroid into hibernation mode. For this reason, I sometimes advise my clients to give up fasting and instead eat smaller portions in the evening. Again, it's best to consult a healthcare provider or nutritionist for personalised advice, as the benefits of fasting should be weighed up against the potential impact on your hormones.

Hormone Supportive Foods

Diet can play a role in managing the symptoms of perimenopause and supporting overall health.

Beneficial foods for perimenopause:

- **Turmeric:** Turmeric contains curcumin, which has anti-inflammatory properties and may help alleviate joint pain and inflammation, common during perimenopause.
- **Saffron:** Saffron may have mood-lifting properties and can help manage mood swings and irritability, which can be associated with hormonal fluctuations.
- **Avocado:** Avocado provides healthy monounsaturated fats, which can support hormone production and overall wellbeing.
- **Maca Powder:** Maca is believed to help balance hormones naturally and may alleviate symptoms like hot flushes and mood swings.
- **Dandelion Root:** Dandelion root tea can support liver health, aiding in hormonal balance and potentially reducing bloating and fluid retention.
- **Flaxseeds and Linseeds:** Flaxseeds are rich in lignans may help manage hormonal imbalances. They are also a source of omega-3 fatty acids.
- **Hemp Seeds:** Hemp seeds are high in omega-3 fatty acids and protein, which can help with hormonal balance and overall health.

- **Cauliflower:** Cauliflower can support liver detoxification, potentially helping with hormone metabolism.
- **Nori:** Nori seaweed is a source of iodine, which is important for thyroid health during perimenopause.
- **Kefir and Natural Yoghurt:** These fermented dairy products provide probiotics that support gut health. A healthy gut microbiome can influence hormonal balance and overall wellbeing.
- **Pumpkin Seeds and Sesame Seeds:** These seeds are rich in zinc, which is essential for hormonal regulation and immune function.
- **Cocoa/Cacao:** These contain magnesium, which can help with mood swings and irritability, common during perimenopause.
- **Seafood:** Seafood, particularly fatty fish, provides omega-3 fatty acids, which can help with inflammation and hormonal balance.
- **Lean Protein:** Lean protein sources like poultry and fish are important for muscle maintenance and overall health during perimenopause.
- **Legumes and pulses:** Legumes like beans and lentils provide plant-based protein, fibre and nutrients that support energy levels and overall health.
- **Almonds and Macadamia Nuts:** These nuts offer healthy fats, vitamins and minerals, contributing to hormonal balance and overall wellbeing.
- **Leafy Greens:** Leafy greens are rich in vitamins, minerals and antioxidants that support overall health and may help with mood and energy levels.
- **Berries, Papaya, Pineapple, Apples, Pears, Capsicum, Tomatoes:** These fruits and vegetables provide vitamins, fibre and antioxidants that support overall health and may help manage weight and inflammation.
- **Extra-Virgin Olive Oil:** EVOO is a source of healthy fats and antioxidants that support overall health.

Individual responses to foods can vary, so it's essential to listen to your body and adjust your diet as needed. If you have specific dietary restrictions or medical conditions, consult a healthcare provider, registered nutritionist or dietitian for personalised advice on managing perimenopausal symptoms and supporting your overall health.

Perimenopause 7-Day Sample Meal Plan

	Day 1	Day 2	Day 3	Day 4	Day 5	Day 6	Day 7
Upon waking	Lemon juice or apple cider vinegar in warm water	Lemon juice or apple cider vinegar in warm water	Lemon juice or apple cider vinegar in warm water	Lemon juice or apple cider vinegar in warm water	Lemon juice or apple cider vinegar in warm water	Lemon juice or apple cider vinegar in warm water	Lemon juice or apple cider vinegar in warm water
Breakfast	Green Vanilla Smoothie (p. 108)	Blue Pea Breakfast Bowl with Maple Nut Granola (p. 138)	Green Vanilla Smoothie (p. 108)	Turmeric Chia Berry Pudding (p. 123) + yoghurt	Turmeric Chia Berry Pudding (p. 123) + yoghurt	Collagen Breakfast Smoothie (p. 110)	Lemon Poppy Seed Protein Pancakes (p. 286)
Snack (optional)	Gluten-Free Strawberry & Hazelnut Muffins (p. 284)	Zucchini & Chickpea Hummus (p. 266) with veggie sticks and seed crackers	Leftover Gluten-Free Strawberry & Hazelnut Muffins	Roasted Beetroot & Hemp Seed Hummus (p. 250) on corn thins with a sprinkle of feta	Leftover Roasted Beetroot & Hemp Seed Hummus with veggie sticks and seed crackers	Handful of raw nuts/seeds and a piece of fruit	Corn thins topped with avocado and tomato
Lunch	Fennel Detox Salad Bowl with Black Bean Hummus (p. 164)	Leftover Fennel Detox Salad Bowl with Black Bean Hummus	Egg Nutty Lunch Bowl with Creamy Avocado Dressing (p. 156)	Salad and avocado wrap with your protein of choice	Salad and avocado wrap with your protein of choice	Mushroom & Mozzarella Stacks with Pesto (p. 147)	Leftover Mushroom & Mozzarella Stacks with Pesto
Snack (optional)	Unsweetened yoghurt with berries and nuts/seeds	Leftover Gluten-Free Strawberry & Hazelnut Muffins	Leftover Zucchini & Chickpea Hummus with veggie sticks and seed crackers	Unsweetened yoghurt with berries and nuts/seeds	Unsweetened yoghurt with berries and nuts/seeds	Corn thins topped with avocado and tomato	Handful of raw nuts/seeds and a piece of fruit
Dinner	Lamb & Macadamia Red Curry with Cauliflower Rice (p. 213) V: chickpeas or tofu	Chickpea, Tofu & Spinach Pasta (p. 235)	Spelt Gnocchi with Rich Tomato Sauce (p. 234)	Chicken Thighs with Mushroom Sauce (p. 226) + leafy salad and freekeh V: tofu	Quick Tomato, Walnut & Chickpea Stew (p. 218)	Baked Seafood and Halloumi Parcels (p. 227) + steamed veggies and roasted sweet potato	Spaghetti with Mushroom & Tofu Balls (p. 222)
Supper (optional)	Herbal tea and 2 squares of dark chocolate	Lemon Hemp Bliss Balls (p. 287)	Mango, Pawpaw & Pear Fruit Salad with Banana Sauce & Roasted Coconut (p. 283)	Herbal tea and a low-GI piece of fruit	Herbal tea and 2 squares of dark chocolate	Leftover Lemon Hemp Bliss Balls	Leftover Mango, Pawpaw & Pear Fruit Salad with Banana Sauce & Roasted Coconut

Case Study – Perimenopause

Catherine is 43 years old, married and has a 12-year-old daughter. She works full-time and is often on the road seeing clients, so she lacks routine and is very busy and stressed. She often wakes through the night in a panic and has trouble getting back to sleep. She is over the healthy weight range for her height.

Catherine explained that she feels generally depressed and anxious and cries easily. She experiences constant bloating, sugar cravings, mild hot flushes and reflux, particularly when she drinks alcohol or too much coffee. Her menstrual cycle is heavy and erratic; her sex drive is low. She does not exercise but does intermittent fasting from 7 pm to 10 am the next day, when she typically has her first meal of the day.

She loves food and eats pretty much everything, but she is prone to overeating, likes sugary foods and does not drink enough water during the day. She has also got into the habit of drinking two or three glasses of wine each night, while she is making dinner.

Nutrition

I started Catherine on a two-week cleanse, to kickstart her liver function. This meant eliminating a wide range of items from her diet: red meat, pork, caffeinated drinks, soft drinks, alcohol, foods containing gluten or dairy (including bread and pasta), white rice, cooked oils, bottled products (even tomato sauces!), tinned/canned foods and processed foods.

From there, we implemented an ongoing food program that included a variety of fruits, vegetables, gluten-free whole grains, lean proteins and healthy fats.

We also adjusted Catherine's diet by:

- reducing her intake of high-GI foods and making sure she had good-quality protein and good fats with every meal and snack, which reduced the insulin spikes she had been experiencing and kept her feeling fuller for longer
- incorporating foods rich in calcium (leafy greens, dairy products, fortified plant-based milk) and vitamin D (fatty fish, egg yolks, fortified foods) to support her bone health
- increasing her consumption of foods rich in phytoestrogens, such as soy products, flaxseeds, sesame seeds, chickpeas, lentils and other legumes*

- stopping her intermittent fasting. Instead, I suggested that she eat smaller portions at night. Catherine responded well to these dietary adjustments, started losing weight and discovered that her perimenopausal symptoms began to subside.

These foods may benefit some women and make symptoms worse for others. Always consult a healthcare provider or nutritionist before making any significant changes to your diet.

She now drinks at least two litres of water each day, has switched from coffee to green tea and decaffeinated coffee, cut out carbonated soft drinks altogether and limits her alcoholic drinks to just one or two glasses every second or third day (instead of every day). These tweaks have improved her hydration and hot flushes.

I also recommended that Catherine take the following supplements:

- prebiotics and probiotics, to boost her digestive system
- chromium and milk thistle, to aid her blood sugar levels and support her liver
- methylated vitamin B complex with a focus on vitamins B5 and B6, to reduce stress and keep her hormones in balance
- ashwagandha, curcumin and vitex, which are all natural adaptogenic herbs that have been demonstrated to help with stress hormones such as cortisol and reducing hot flushes and mood swings.

Note: Methylated vitamin B complex supplements contain B vitamins in a form that is considered more bioavailable and easier for the body to absorb and utilise. It depends on an individual's specific needs and genetic factors: some people may benefit more from taking methylated forms due to difficulties in metabolising standard B vitamins, while others may not require methylated versions. As always, consult a healthcare professional for personalised guidance on whether to use methylated B complex supplements.

Note: Adaptogenic herbs are believed to help regulate hormones by supporting the body's natural ability to adapt to stress. When the body encounters stressors, whether physical, emotional, or environmental, the endocrine system responds by releasing hormones like cortisol and adrenaline. Prolonged or excessive stress can disrupt hormonal balance, leading to issues such as adrenal fatigue, thyroid dysfunction and hormonal imbalances in women. Adaptogens are thought to modulate the body's stress response, reducing the overproduction of stress hormones and helping to normalise hormone levels. By promoting this balance, adaptogenic herbs may contribute to overall hormonal health and alleviate symptoms related to hormonal imbalances, such as fatigue, mood swings and irregular menstrual cycles. However, more research is needed to fully understand the mechanisms by which adaptogens influence hormonal regulation.

Movement

Catherine is now doing regular strength-based physical activity for at least 30 minutes each session, most days of the week. She has started going to the local dancing studio, which she finds really fun, and she has also taken up yoga, walking, jogging and swimming.

Mind

Catherine has been practising stress-reducing deep-breathing techniques. She finds this therapeutic and easy to do anytime and anywhere. She goes to bed earlier and aims for seven to nine hours of quality sleep each night. To facilitate this, she has created a relaxing bedtime routine, playing calming music, turning the light down and following a strict no-screen rule for at least 90 minutes before bed. She is using a sleep tracker app, too, to monitor her slumber patterns and disruptions.

Catherine has also begun seeing a psychotherapist, who has given her tools to identify and manage her anxiety and depression. These include reframing her thoughts and internal dialogue to be more positive, and tips for how to 'break the cycle' quickly.

Mantra – Fall in love with the journey, while striving towards the destination.

Connection

Catherine recently joined a book club, whose members are mainly women around her age and with similar interests to her. When they come together, these women not only discuss the specific book they are reading but also share their day-to-day experiences, including their experiences of going through perimenopause or menopause. Catherine has found it very therapeutic to be part of this group and receive emotional support from others undergoing the same transition as she is.

Conventional Medicine

On my recommendation, Catherine saw her GP for a blood test to assess her hormone levels, including her thyroid function and antibodies. Thyroid symptoms and perimenopausal symptoms can often overlap, leading to confusion and misdiagnosis. Both conditions share common signs such as fatigue, mood swings, weight changes and irregular menstrual cycles. This similarity occurs because thyroid hormones play a crucial role in regulating the menstrual cycle, and thyroid dysfunction can disrupt hormonal balance. Additionally, both perimenopause and thyroid issues can lead to sleep disturbances, anxiety and cognitive changes. It's essential for women experiencing these symptoms, especially those in their late 30s to early 50s, to consult a healthcare professional who can conduct thorough evaluations, including thyroid function tests and hormone assessments, to differentiate between the two conditions. Accurate diagnosis is vital for appropriate treatment and management of either thyroid disorders or perimenopause symptoms.

When she received the results, her thyroid function was within normal range, but there were irregularities in her levels of progesterone, oestradiol, luteinising hormone (LH), follicle stimulating hormone (FSH) and sex hormone–binding globulin (SHBG) – indicating that she might be perimenopausal. Her morning cortisol (stress hormone) level was elevated, as was her morning glucose, indicating she was likely insulin resistant.

For her general health, she also did a full blood count – looking at white and red blood cells, liver function, kidney function, inflammation, blood glucose, zinc and cholesterol.

Note: For more information on how hormones can affect thyroid function, see the 'Hormones and Thyroid Health' chapter.

Overall, Catherine's perimenopausal symptoms have diminished: she is feeling less depressed and anxious, sleeping better, and feels more knowledgeable, empowering her to make health-related choices that are right for her at this life stage, and to talk about them more openly.

Menopause

Although I am yet to experience menopause myself, I remember watching my mother transition from perimenopause to menopause. When my mother was perimenopausal, she seemed to turn into a different woman: one who was often overwhelmed and would lose her temper at the drop of a hat. I also remember thinking to myself then, *I don't ever want to go through that.*

Looking back, I now have a huge amount of empathy for her, as she was really struggling with her perimenopausal symptoms. She tried hormone replacement therapy (HRT), exercise and natural remedies ... but nothing provided sustained relief. She seldom talked about what she was going through but I now understand how very alone and confused she must have felt then.

Menopause is a natural and inevitable phase in a woman's life, marking the end of the menstrual cycle and reproductive years. While the average age of menopause is around 51, it can occur anywhere between the ages of 45 and 55, and in rare cases, even earlier or later. This transition is characterised by a significant shift in hormonal balance, with key sex hormones undergoing notable changes.

It's easy to focus on the negatives, but there are many benefits to this transition. There's the obvious one of bidding farewell to monthly periods, of course. No more need for tampons, pads, or dealing with menstrual cramps! Since fertility declines significantly during menopause, many women can also stop using contraceptives, if their concern was falling pregnant, but still it's worthwhile noting they are important to protect women against STIs. But it can give them more freedom and choice in their sex lives. And talking about sex, there are so many brilliant and natural lubrication products on the market which can help with vaginal dryness.

Some women experience improved sleep during menopause, as they no longer have to contend with the night sweats and hot flushes that can disrupt rest. You may experience fewer mood swings, too, as your hormones are more stable.

Menopause can bring relief to women who've struggled with endometriosis, as oestrogen levels fall, leading to a decrease in the painful symptoms associated with this condition. It can also alleviate the symptoms of polycystic ovary syndrome (PCOS).

While menopause itself is not a guarantee against cancer, decreased exposure to oestrogen can reduce the risk of uterine and ovarian cancers.

Menopause often marks a life transition. With the challenges of menstruation behind, many women use this time to focus on self-care, pursue new hobbies or explore new interests.

Hormonal changes during menopause

Hormone Levels

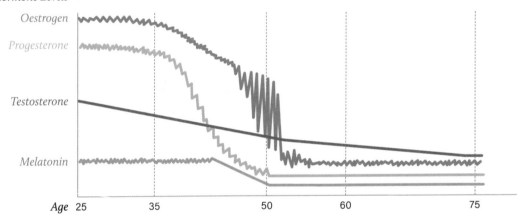

This graph shows the dramatic hormonal crash that women experience during menopause. Let's explore the specific hormones involved, and the effects of their decline on the mind and body.

- **Oestrogen:** One of the most prominent changes during menopause is the decline in oestrogen levels. Oestrogen, a hormone produced primarily by the ovaries, plays a vital role in regulating the menstrual cycle, maintaining bone density and supporting vaginal health. As menopause approaches, the ovaries produce less oestrogen, leading to a range of physical and emotional changes, such as hot flushes, night sweats, vaginal dryness, joint pain, changes to hair and skin, weight gain, sleep disruptions, anxiety, depression, fatigue, memory changes and mood swings.
- **Progesterone:** Progesterone, another hormone produced by the ovaries, also declines. This hormone is responsible for preparing the uterine lining for pregnancy each month. Its levels drop as menopause sets in, contributing to irregular menstrual cycles and affecting mood and sleep patterns.

- **Testosterone:** While often associated with males, testosterone is also present in females, albeit in smaller amounts. Testosterone supports libido, energy levels and overall wellbeing. During menopause, testosterone levels can decrease, leading to reduced sex drive and energy.
- **Melatonin:** This hormone regulates the sleep–wake cycle and is produced in the brain's pineal gland. Changes in estrogen levels can lower melatonin production, potentially impacting the ability to fall asleep and the overall quality of sleep.

Menopausal symptoms

The hormonal changes that occur during menopause can give rise to a host of symptoms that impact a woman's physical and emotional wellbeing. Some common symptoms of menopause include:

- **Hot flushes:** Hot flushes are sudden waves of intense heat and sweating, often accompanied by a flushed face and neck.
- **Night sweats:** Night sweats are like hot flushes but occur during sleep, leading to disrupted rest.
- **Weight gain:** Changes in hormonal balance can contribute to weight gain, particularly around the abdominal area.
- **Sleep disturbances:** Fluctuations in hormones can lead to difficulties falling asleep or staying asleep.
- **Mood swings:** Hormonal changes can impact neurotransmitters, leading to mood swings, irritability, depression and anxiety.
- **Vaginal dryness:** Declining oestrogen levels can result in vaginal dryness and discomfort.
- **Low libido:** Reduced testosterone levels can lead to a decreased interest in sexual activity.
- **Urinary incontinence:** Changes in pelvic floor muscles and vaginal tissues can lead to bladder control issues.
- **Sexual pain:** Vaginal dryness and thinning tissues can cause discomfort during intercourse.
- **Joint pain:** Oestrogen aids in the production of lubricating fluid and reduces inflammation, so decreasing oestrogen levels can result in pain in the joints.

Diagnosis

It's important to note that low thyroid hormone levels can cause symptoms like those of menopause. Fatigue, mood changes, weight gain and sleep disturbances can be attributed to both menopause and hypothyroidism. Moreover, low oestrogen levels can impact thyroid hormone production, potentially exacerbating menopausal symptoms. Your GP or medical specialist can order blood tests to check your hormone levels. The tests they ask for will depend on the symptoms you are experiencing. The most common baseline blood tests requested for menopause are outlined in the table below.

Menopause	Thyroid Function	Cortisol
Luteinising hormone (LH)	TSH	DHEA
Follicle stimulating hormone (FSH)	Free T4	Cortisol
E2 (oestradiol)	Free T3	ACTH
Progesterone	Reverse T3	
Sex hormone–binding globulin (SHBG)	Thyroid antibodies (TPOAbs and TgAbs)	
Iron		
Vitamin D3	Zinc	
Total cholesterol	Iodine	
Trigs	Selenium	
HDL	Iron	
LDL		
Diabetes – fasting blood sugar, HbA1c, glucose tolerance test		

There are also functional tests available that will give you a further picture of your hormonal health, including urinary cortisol, urinary iodine, urinary hormone and saliva testing for cortisol and sex hormones.

Managing menopausal symptoms

Other ways to manage menopausal symptoms often involve a multifaceted approach that addresses both hormonal changes and individual needs. Here are some strategies to consider:

- **Lifestyle modifications:** Regular exercise, a balanced diet rich in nutrients, and stress-reduction techniques can help alleviate symptoms and support overall wellbeing.
- **Vaginal moisturisers and lubricants:** These can provide relief from vaginal dryness and discomfort during intercourse.

- **Pelvic floor exercises:** Strengthening pelvic floor muscles can help manage urinary incontinence.
- **Hormone replacement therapy (HRT):** This involves supplementing the body with hormones like oestrogen and progesterone to alleviate symptoms. The decision to pursue HRT should only be made after discussing the potential benefits and risks with a healthcare provider.
- **Medications:** Medications can be prescribed to manage specific symptoms, such as mood swings, sleep disturbances and hot flushes.

Hormone Supportive Foods

In addition to the strategies mentioned above, there are several foods that can help balance hormones and alleviate symptoms during menopause. Including these hormone-supportive foods in your diet can be beneficial:

- **Soy Products:** Soy contains phytoestrogens and isoflavones, which mimic the effects of oestrogen in the body. Incorporating tofu, tempeh, soy milk and edamame into your diet may help alleviate some menopausal symptoms. (It's important to note, though, that some women may be sensitive to phytoestrogens and experience adverse effects. It's best to consult a healthcare provider or nutritionist before making any changes, because you may need to limit your intake of certain phytoestrogens rather than increasing your intake.)
- **Flaxseeds:** Flaxseeds are rich in lignans, which have oestrogenic properties. They may help balance hormone levels and reduce hot flushes. Ground flaxseeds can be added to smoothies, yoghurt or oatmeal.
- **Fatty Fish:** Fatty fish like salmon, mackerel and sardines are high in omega-3 fatty acids, which can help reduce inflammation and support heart health. They may also have a positive effect on mood swings and cognitive function.
- **Leafy Greens:** Dark, leafy greens such as spinach, kale and silverbeet are packed with vitamins and minerals, including calcium and magnesium, which are essential for bone health during menopause.
- **Nuts and Seeds:** Almonds, walnuts, pumpkin seeds and sunflower seeds are good sources of healthy fats, fibre and vitamin E. They can help combat weight gain and support skin and hair health.
- **Whole Grains:** Opt for whole grains like quinoa, brown rice and whole wheat over refined grains. These provide sustained energy and fibre, which can aid in managing weight and digestive health.

- **Dairy or Dairy Alternatives:** Low-fat dairy or fortified dairy alternatives like almond milk can provide calcium and vitamin D for bone health.
- **Berries:** Berries, such as blueberries and strawberries, are rich in antioxidants and can support cognitive function and overall health.
- **Cruciferous Vegetables:** Vegetables like broccoli, cauliflower and brussels sprouts contain compounds that support liver detoxification and hormone balance.
- **Herbal Teas:** Herbal teas like chamomile, peppermint and black cohosh tea may help alleviate hot flushes and promote relaxation.
- **Protein Sources:** Lean sources of protein like lean poultry, lamb, beef, seafood and other vegetarian proteins like beans, lentils and quinoa can help maintain muscle mass and support energy levels.
- **Water:** Staying well hydrated is essential to manage hot flushes and maintain overall health. Drinking plenty of water can also support urinary tract health.
- **Sage:** Sage may help reduce hot flushes and night sweats, common symptoms during menopause, although more research is needed to confirm its effectiveness.
- **Citrus Fruit (Lemons, Oranges, Limes, Grapefruits):** Citrus fruits are rich in vitamin C and other antioxidants, which support immune function and overall health.

Foods to limit or avoid during menopause:

- **Excessive Caffeine and Alcohol:** High caffeine and alcohol consumption can disrupt sleep patterns, exacerbate hot flushes and contribute to mood swings.
- **Spicy Foods:** Spicy foods can trigger or worsen hot flushes in some women.
- **Highly Processed Foods:** Processed foods, sugary snacks and high-sugar beverages can lead to weight gain and contribute to mood swings and fatigue.
- **Salty Foods:** Excess sodium can lead to bloating and exacerbate water retention, which may already be an issue during menopause.
- **Fried and Fatty Foods:** High-fat foods can contribute to weight gain and may worsen symptoms like mood swings and irritability.

It's important to maintain a balanced diet that includes nutrient-rich foods to support overall health and manage menopausal symptoms effectively. Staying hydrated, engaging in regular physical activity and managing stress are also crucial components of a healthy lifestyle during menopause. Consult with a healthcare provider or registered dietitian for personalised guidance on managing menopause through diet and lifestyle adjustments.

Menopause 7-Day Sample Meal Plan

	Day 1	Day 2	Day 3	Day 4	Day 5	Day 6	Day 7
Upon waking	Lemon juice or apple cider vinegar in warm water	Lemon juice or apple cider vinegar in warm water	Lemon juice or apple cider vinegar in warm water	Lemon juice or apple cider vinegar in warm water	Lemon juice or apple cider vinegar in warm water	Lemon juice or apple cider vinegar in warm water	Lemon juice or apple cider vinegar in warm water
Breakfast	Collagen Breakfast Smoothie (p. 110)	Collagen Breakfast Smoothie (p. 110)	Lemon & Coconut Buckwheat Porridge (p. 118)	Blue Pea Breakfast Bowl with Maple Nut Granola (p. 138)	Miso Mushroom Scrambled Eggs (p. 142)	Turmeric Chia Berry Pudding (p. 123) + yoghurt	Acai Berry & Chocolate Soufflé Sweet Omelette (p. 276)
Snack (optional)	Unsweetened yoghurt with berries and LSA	Leftover Avocado Edamame Hummus with veggie sticks	Handful of raw nuts/ seeds and a piece of fruit	Pumpkin & Banana Brown Rice Muffins with Strawberries (p. 291)	Leftover Macadamia Nut Pâté with veggie sticks	Leftover Pumpkin & Banana Brown Rice Muffins with Strawberries	Unsweetened yoghurt with berries and LSA
Lunch	Dairy-Free Pesto, Potato & Egg Salad (p. 186)	Turmeric, Sicilian Olive & Parmesan Loaf (p. 195), topped with avocado + a side salad	Leftover Turmeric, Sicilian Olive & Parmesan Loaf, topped with avocado + a side salad	Chilled Beetroot Soup (p. 178) with seeded toast	Leftover Chilled Beetroot Soup with seeded toast	Chickpea & Quinoa Greek Salad (p. 165)	Warm Roasted Vegetable Salad with Tahini Coriander Beetroot Dressing (p. 148) + halloumi, tofu, canned salmon or tuna
Snack (optional)	Avocado Edamame Hummus (p. 154) with veggie sticks	Unsweetened yoghurt with berries and LSA	Unsweetened yoghurt with berries and LSA	Macadamia Nut Pâté (p. 254) with veggie sticks	Unsweetened yoghurt with berries and LSA	Leftover Macadamia Nut Pâté with veggie sticks	Handful of raw nuts/seeds and a piece of fruit
Dinner	Baked Barramundi with Honey Carrots (p. 201) V: pan-fried tofu	Green Curry with Tofu, Peas & Capsicum (p. 212)	Mushroom & Sweet Potato Shepherd's Pie (p. 228)	Roasted Cauliflower Salad with Spiced Almond Butter Dressing (p. 223)	Chicken Biryani with Coconut Yoghurt Dressing (p. 204) V: mushrooms	Cashew-Crumbed Salmon Lettuce Cups (p. 199) + optional steamed brown rice V: tofu	Meatballs with Zucchini & Parmesan Salad (p. 209) V: veggie patty
Supper (optional)	Homemade Chocolate Nut Coconut Bars (p. 285)	Herbal tea and 2 squares of dark chocolate	Lemon Hemp Bliss Balls (p. 287)	Mango, Pawpaw & Pear Fruit Salad with Banana Sauce and Roasted Coconut (p. 283)	Herbal tea with 2–5 macadamias	½ Gluten-Free Strawberry and Hazelnut Muffin (p. 284)	Herbal tea with berries

Case Study – Menopause

Olivia is 52 years old and in a high-stress job. She is also married, a mother of two young adults who still live at home, and has older parents who rely on her for support in much of their day-to-day life. She approached me with worsening hormonal symptoms, hot flushes, poor digestion, low sex drive and weight gain. She had recently had her gall bladder removed, and, when we did her blood test, her C-reactive protein was elevated, which is an indicator of inflammation. Her bone density was lower than average. She also experiences frequent bloating, and her bowel movements often alternate between constipation and diarrhoea. She makes time for daily exercise, which has been her saving grace. She has had a contraceptive intrauterine device (IUD) for 20 years and has not had a period for a few years.

Nutrition

I started Olivia on a two-week cleanse, to detox her liver. We eliminated a wide range of items from her diet: red meat, pork, caffeinated drinks, soft drinks, alcohol, foods containing gluten or dairy (including bread and pasta), white rice, cooked oils, bottled products (even tomato sauces!), tinned/canned foods and processed foods.

From there, we implemented an ongoing food program that included a variety of fruits, vegetables, gluten-free whole grains, lean proteins and healthy fats.

We also adjusted Olivia's diet by:

- increasing her intake of foods rich in calcium and vitamin D, to support her bone density
- limiting caffeine, alcohol and processed foods, as they were exacerbating her hormonal imbalances and symptoms
- adding phytoestrogen-rich foods like soy, flaxseeds and chickpeas to her diet, to help alleviate her symptoms (it's important to note, though, that some women may be sensitive to phytoestrogens and experience adverse effects; it's best to consult a healthcare provider or nutritionist before making any changes, because you may need to limit your intake of certain phytoestrogens rather than increasing your intake)
- identifying and eliminating foods that were triggering her symptoms, which turned out to be gluten, dairy, caffeine and spicy foods.

Olivia keeps a food journal now and tracks her symptoms, so she can identify triggers and make informed choices about what she eats.

Over the course of working with Olivia for six months, I suggested the following supplements:

- probiotics, to support a healthy gut microbiome
- high-strength turmeric (curcumin) and saffron, to help with inflammation and mood
- calcium and vitamin D, for bone health
- omega-3 fatty acids, for heart health
- magnesium, to support muscle and nerve function
- milk thistle, for liver support.

Movement

Olivia was already exercising regularly, but she mainly did high-intensity exercise, which can exacerbate cortisol levels, working counterproductively against weight loss. We incorporated a mix of aerobic exercise (brisk walking, swimming and cycling) and strength training for muscle health and bone density. She also incorporated Bikram yoga (a form of yoga that takes place in a heated environment) into her exercise regimen, and now goes for fortnightly ice baths and infrared saunas, which increase blood flow and oxygen to the brain, boosting her mood and reducing the stress hormone cortisol – all of which are having a positive impact on her stress levels and flexibility.

Mind

In addition to Bikram yoga, Olivia has been practising meditation to alleviate her stress and promote better sleep. She prefers a 'yoga nidra' style meditation to wind down most evenings before sleep and usually picks a guided practice from the wide selection available on the meditation app Insight Timer.

Olivia has also been reading a book called *The Reality Slap* by Dr Russ Harris, a renowned acceptance and commitment therapy (ACT) trainer and author. The book provides scientifically proven tips and techniques for coping effectively with issues in life, which she has been using whenever she is feeling stressed or anxious.

Mantra – Health is fluid, take the good with the bad and know that this too shall pass.

Connection

Olivia joined a series of 'laughter yoga' workshops. Laughter yoga is a unique practice that combines laughter exercises with yogic breathing techniques, often in a group setting. She is finding these sessions therapeutic: they improve her mood and help her to relax and cope with stress.

Conventional Medicine

When Olivia came to see me, she was already on oestrogen-replacement therapy, as advised by her GP. For a complete picture of her hormone profile, I recommended she go for a DUTCH urine test (dried urine test for comprehensive hormones). The results showed that her oestrogen levels were low even for a menopausal woman, supporting her GP's advice that she try oestrogen-replacement therapy.

Olivia is loving the new foods that we introduced into her diet. She is being more creative with her meals and has noticed that she has lost weight, her moods are more stable and she's having fewer hot flushes. She has also noticed that the supplements and changes to her exercise regimen have made her feel calmer and stronger and further helped with her weight.

Postmenopause

My late maternal grandmother was a very stoic woman and never talked about anything to do with her feminine health, which she would have considered taboo. As a result, I have no clue how menopause affected her, or how her postmenopause life was different. Lucky for us, times change – we are much more open about female health today, and I look forward to sharing my experiences and knowledge of this important transition with my grandchildren in the future.

Postmenopause is the phase of a woman's life after menopause. During this time, hormones are still adjusting, so some women continue to experience symptoms of menopause, whereas symptoms will ease or stop for other women and finally stabilise.

As oestrogen levels drop during menopause and then remain at a lower level during postmenopause, adrenal DHEA becomes one of the major precursors of estrogens and androgens. This means supporting adrenal gland function is really important.

Oestrogen's protective effect on heart and blood vessel health is diminished postmenopause, and decreased oestrogen is also associated with increased total body fat, especially around the abdominal area. Menopause and postmenopause can therefore increase a woman's risk of cardiovascular disease and also metabolic syndrome. This makes weight management, blood sugar control and cardiovascular disease risk management important focus areas. Additionally, due to the drop in oestrogen and the reduction in bone density, menopausal and postmenopausal women are at increased risk of osteoporosis.

Hormonal changes stabilise postmenopause, but sleep disruptions may still be an issue: some women may still have the occasional hot flush or night sweat, so it's important to focus on healthy sleep hygiene.

After menopause, women benefit from a diet that not only helps manage ongoing hormonal changes such as healthy blood sugar levels but also addresses specific health concerns like those I've just mentioned. Here are some foods that can be helpful during postmenopause.

Hormone Supportive Foods

With their heightened risk of cardiovascular disease and osteoporosis, postmenopausal women should eat foods that support a healthy heart, bones and blood vessels, such as:

- **Calcium-Rich Foods:** Adequate calcium intake is crucial for maintaining bone health and preventing osteoporosis. Include dairy products, fortified plant-based milk alternatives, greens (e.g. kale, bok choy), almonds and canned salmon or sardines (with bones) in your diet.
- **Vitamin D:** Vitamin D is essential for calcium absorption and bone health. Fatty fish like salmon and mackerel, fortified dairy or plant-based milk, egg yolks and spending time in the sun can help increase vitamin D levels.
- **Fibre-Rich Foods:** High-fibre foods like whole grains, legumes (beans, lentils), vegetables and fruits can aid in weight management, support healthy digestion and help stabilise blood sugar levels.
- **Omega-3 Fatty Acids:** Foods rich in omega-3 fatty acids, such as fatty fish (salmon, trout), walnuts, flaxseeds and chia seeds, can reduce inflammation and support cardiovascular health.
- **Lean Proteins:** Lean sources of protein like poultry, fish, tofu and legumes can help maintain muscle mass and support weight management.
- **Antioxidant-Rich Foods:** Antioxidants help protect the heart and blood vessels. Include berries (blueberries, strawberries), citrus fruits, nuts and dark chocolate (in moderation) in your diet.
- **Healthy Fats:** Include sources of healthy fats in your diet, such as fatty fish (rich in omega-3 fatty acids), nuts, seeds, extra-virgin olive oil and avocado. These fats can help improve heart health.
- **Adaptogenic Herbs:** Some adaptogenic herbs, such as ashwagandha and rhodiola, can help support adrenal gland function. Consult a healthcare provider before using herbal supplements.
- **Low–Glycaemic Index Foods:** Choosing foods with a low glycaemic index, like whole grains, legumes and non-starchy vegetables, can help manage blood sugar levels and reduce the risk of metabolic syndrome.
- **Spices and Herbs:** Turmeric, cinnamon and garlic have anti-inflammatory properties and can contribute to heart health.
- **Green Tea:** Green tea contains antioxidants and has been associated with improved cardiovascular health.

- **Probiotic Foods:** Yoghurt, kefir, sauerkraut and other probiotic-rich foods can support digestive health and may have indirect benefits for weight management and overall wellbeing.
- **Vitamin K:** Vitamin K plays a significant role in bone health by aiding in calcium absorption and bone mineralisation. Include foods rich in vitamin K, like leafy greens, liver, chicken, egg yolks and tempeh in your diet.
- **Magnesium:** Magnesium is essential for bone density, and it works synergistically with calcium. Incorporate magnesium-rich foods like leafy greens, nuts, seeds, legumes and whole grains to support bone health.
- **Insoluble Fibre:** Insoluble fibre helps the body to assimilate calcium and magnesium. Include foods like wheat bran, oat bran, legumes, green peas, quinoa, leafy greens and almonds in your diet to boost insoluble fibre intake.
- **Dietary Fibre:** Consume more dietary fibre from sources like whole grains, vegetables, legumes, fruits and nuts/seeds. Fibre can help lower cholesterol levels and support heart health.

Remember that overall dietary choices and lifestyle factors, including regular physical activity and stress management, play a significant role in promoting both bone health and cardiovascular health. It's advisable to work with a healthcare provider or registered nutritionist or dietitian to develop a personalised nutrition plan that addresses your specific health concerns and goals.

Postmenopause 7-Day Sample Meal Plan

	Day 1	Day 2	Day 3	Day 4	Day 5	Day 6	Day 7
Upon waking	Lemon juice or apple cider vinegar in warm water	Lemon juice or apple cider vinegar in warm water	Lemon juice or apple cider vinegar in warm water	Lemon juice or apple cider vinegar in warm water	Lemon juice or apple cider vinegar in warm water	Lemon juice or apple cider vinegar in warm water	Lemon juice or apple cider vinegar in warm water
Breakfast	Antioxidant Matcha Cacao Smoothie (p. 109)	Lemon & Coconut Buckwheat Porridge (p. 118)	Turmeric Chia Berry Pudding (p. 123)	Lemon & Coconut Buckwheat Porridge (p. 118)	Zesty Trout, Walnut, Avocado & Lime Salsa Bruschetta (p. 144)	Savoury French Toast with Mushrooms, Goat Cheese and Spirulina Pesto (p. 140)	Roasted Pear, Berries, Hemp & Coconut (p. 135)
Snack	Unsweetened yoghurt with berries and LSA	Cottage cheese and tomato on rice cakes or buckwheat cakes V: avocado	Unsweetened yoghurt with berries and LSA	Turmeric, Walnut & Sweet Potato Dip (p. 253) with veggie sticks and seed crackers	Unsweetened yoghurt with berries and LSA	Leftover Turmeric, Walnut & Sweet Potato Dip with veggie sticks and seed crackers	Berry & Beetroot Smoothie (p. 107)
Lunch	Sweet Potato Noodle Salad with Creamy Cashew & Chia Seeds (p. 150)	Leftover Sweet Potato Noodle Salad with Creamy Cashew & Chia Seeds	Crushed Pea Bruschetta with Avocado & Goat's Cheese Salsa (p. 185)	Prawn, Watermelon & Cashew Lettuce Cups with Coconut Avocado Dressing (p. 188)	Roasted Capsicum & Almond Soup (p. 191)	Leftover Roasted Capsicum & Almond Soup	Broccolini, Brazil Nut & Quinoa Salad with Crispy Halloumi (p. 158) V: tofu
Snack (optional)	Cottage cheese and tomato on rice cakes or buckwheat cakes V: avocado	Unsweetened yoghurt with berries and LSA	Berry & Beetroot Smoothie (p. 107)	Unsweetened yoghurt with berries and LSA	Leftover Turmeric, Walnut & Sweet Potato Dip with veggie sticks and seed crackers	Unsweetened yoghurt with berries and LSA	Unsweetened yoghurt with berries and LSA
Dinner	Warm Ginger Satay Chicken Salad with Turmeric Cauliflower (p. 206) V: chickpeas	Roasted Salmon & Eggplant Poke Plate (p. 224) V: veggie patty	Meatballs with Zucchini & Parmesan Salad (p. 209) V: tofu	Grilled fish with Orange, Goat's Cheese, Almond & Quinoa Salad (p. 260) V: tofu or veggie patty	Spelt Gnocchi with Rich Tomato Sauce (p. 234)	Mushroom & Sweet Potato Shepherd's Pie (p. 228)	Leftover Mushroom & Sweet Potato Shepherd's Pie
Supper (optional)	Herbal tea and 2 squares of dark chocolate	Chocolate & Coconut-Dipped Frozen Fruit (p. 282)	Chai Spiced Apple Crumble with Honey Cinnamon Yoghurt (p. 281)	Lemon Hemp Bliss Balls (p. 287)	Herbal tea and 2 squares of dark chocolate	½ Cacao Beet Brownie (p. 279)	Herbal tea and berries

Case Study – Postmenopausal Woman

Linda is a 60-year-old woman who has transitioned into the postmenopausal phase of her life. She is still working four days a week, which she loves, and has a partner of seven years. Since menopause, Linda has gained a significant amount of weight due to hormonal changes and a slowing metabolism. Her hormonal shifts have led to a decrease in her sex drive and arousal, and vaginal dryness and discomfort, which has affected Linda's intimacy with her partner. She is also experiencing sleep disturbances, which leave her feeling fatigued, and, with her weight gain, low libido and loss of intimacy with her partner, she is feeling low in self-confidence.

Nutrition

I asked Linda to start eating more whole foods, fibre-rich fruits and vegetables and lean proteins, to help her feel fuller for longer, control her weight better and improve her energy levels. We focused on foods high in calcium (such as good-quality dairy products, fortified plant-based milk, leafy greens and almonds) and vitamin D (such as fatty fish and egg yolks). I also suggested that Linda boost her vitamin D by getting more sun.

In terms of supplements, I recommended a probiotic specifically targeting urogenital health and microflora, to help her vaginal dryness and pH levels (to maintain acidity-alkalinity balance). I also added omega-3 fatty acids, to improve her mood and decrease inflammation.

Movement

Linda has started doing tai chi three times a week and walking with friends on the weekends. She has also joined her local yoga studio. These gentle, low-impact activities suit her current level of fitness, helping her to maintain muscle mass and lose weight slowly and sustainably without pushing up her cortisol levels.

Mind

Linda has been using 'Health and Her', which is a perimenopause and menopause symptom tracking app that provides her with free access to expert advice, personalised insights and evidence-based exercises and tools to support her through her current life stage. As a result, she feels more positive about what she is going through and better equipped to cope with the challenges she is facing.

Linda has started seeing a cognitive behavioural therapist and learning techniques to reshape negative thought patterns and work through her emotional concerns, helping to alleviate her self-esteem issues.

She is also doing fortnightly infrared saunas, which have helped boost her mood and decrease stress and inflammation.

Mantra – Find comfort in connection and knowing that the best is yet to come.

Connection

Linda has started volunteering at a homeless shelter, which has elevated her sense of purpose and provided a different perspective on life.

Conventional Medicine

Linda is proactive about keeping on top of her health, visiting her GP regularly for check-ups and getting full blood tests done every six months. This reassures her that all is well and helps her to feel in control.

Linda now feels her physical and emotional wellbeing have improved immensely. She enjoys working with her different healthcare professionals and support networks to find ways to stay healthy and live her best life as she grows older.

Adult Men

For men, young adulthood is a period of exploration, growth and vitality. During this phase they experience their peak testosterone levels, typically between the ages of 20 and 30. Testosterone, often associated with masculine traits, plays a pivotal role in muscle growth, bone health, mood regulation and even libido. At around 30, testosterone starts to fall, which can lead to hormonal imbalances.

Here's what you need to know about testosterone and some of the other primary hormones that can rise and fall over the course of a man's life:

- **Testosterone:** Testosterone is produced mainly in the testicles, under the control of luteinising hormone from the anterior pituitary and a small amount from the adrenal cortex/peripheral tissues.
- **Luteinising Hormone (LH):** LH stimulates production of testosterone.
- **Follicle Stimulating Hormone (FSH):** FSH is necessary for sperm production.
- **Dehydroepiandrosterone (DHEA):** DHEA is the precursor to androgen production, which both decline with age. The body cannot produce testosterone without adequate DHEA.
- **Sex hormone–binding globulin (SHBG):** SHBG is a protein in the blood that binds to certain hormones, including testosterone. SHBG increases with age, resulting in more testosterone being bound and therefore less freely available.
- **Oestradiol:** Oestradiol is a hormone produced from cholesterol and a type of naturally occurring oestrogen.

Navigating the testosterone decline

As the clock ticks, testosterone declines, giving rise to 'andropause'. While the drop is small and gradual, it can trigger symptoms that impact wellbeing, such as fatigue, anxiety, depression and weight gain; it also increases the risk of osteoporosis and can negatively affect your motivation, confidence and libido.

Many factors can exacerbate this testosterone decline. Obesity is one: as you gain weight, more testosterone is converted to oestrogen via the aromatase enzyme. Others are excessive alcohol consumption; a diet high in saturated fats and refined carbohydrates; inflammation; and stress.

Strategies for hormonal harmony

Research suggests a link between low thyroid levels and reduced testosterone production. Stress can affect testosterone production too, so keeping cortisol under control is also important. Understanding the hormonal balance isn't just about knowledge, it's about action. Here are some common problems and strategies for dealing with them:

- **Stress-induced hormonal disruption:** If stress is the culprit behind hormonal imbalances, adopting stress-reduction techniques like deep breathing, meditation and mindfulness can be immensely beneficial. Nutrients like magnesium, zinc and B vitamins can provide support during challenging times.
- **Inflammation and excessive oestrogen conversion:** Oestrogen dominance in men can lead to infertility, overdevelopment of breast tissue, erectile dysfunction and other symptoms. To combat inflammation and the over-conversion of testosterone to oestrogen, focus on reducing body fat percentage. Limiting alcohol intake and incorporating anti-inflammatory and antioxidant-rich foods like salmon, chia or hemp, seeds, turmeric and green tea can contribute to hormonal harmony.
- **Excess xenoestrogens:** Xenoestrogens are compounds that mimic oestrogen and can increase oestrogen levels in the body, leading to similar symptoms of oestrogen dominance. To avoid xenoestrogens, try to minimise your exposure to plastics and pesticides, and increase your intake of phytoestrogens from foods like flaxseed, tempeh, legumes and miso, to help modulate your oestrogen levels.

Hormone Supportive Foods

These foods are beneficial for supporting men's hormonal health due to their nutrient composition and various health-promoting properties:

- **Avocado:** Avocado provides healthy monounsaturated fats that are important for hormone production and overall health.
- **Fatty Fish (Salmon):** Fatty fish like salmon are rich in omega-3 fatty acids, which help regulate hormones and reduce inflammation. Omega-3s are crucial for maintaining healthy testosterone levels.
- **Nuts/Seeds:** Nuts and seeds, such as walnuts, flaxseeds and chia seeds, provide healthy fats, fibre and minerals that support hormone production and overall wellbeing.

- **Extra-Virgin Olive Oil (EVOO):** EVOO contains monounsaturated fats and antioxidants that can positively impact hormone balance and reduce inflammation.
- **Fruits and Vegetables:** A diet rich in a variety of fruits and vegetables provides essential vitamins, minerals, antioxidants and fibre that support overall health and hormone regulation.
- **Cocoa/Cacao:** Cocoa and cacao contain compounds that may have a positive effect on mood and overall hormonal health.
- **Whole Grains:** Whole grains offer complex carbohydrates and fibre that help stabilise blood sugar levels, which is important for hormonal balance and energy.
- **Lean Protein:** Lean sources of protein like fish, chicken, eggs and unsweetened yoghurt provide the building blocks necessary for hormone synthesis and muscle development.
- **Fermented Foods:** Fermented foods like kefir, sauerkraut, kimchi and kombucha support gut health. A healthy gut microbiome can indirectly influence hormonal balance and overall wellbeing.
- **Herbs and Spices:** Many herbs and spices, such as turmeric, have anti-inflammatory properties and can support overall health, including hormonal health.
- **Antioxidant-Rich Foods:** Foods like pomegranates, berries, green tea and turmeric are rich in antioxidants, which can protect cells from oxidative stress – a process that causes cell damage – and potentially support hormonal balance.
- **Phytoestrogens:** Foods like flax, sesame seeds and linseeds contain phytoestrogens, which can help balance oestrogen levels in the body.
- **Honey:** Some research suggests that honey may have a positive effect on testosterone levels.
- **Fenugreek:** Fenugreek is a herb that has been associated with potential benefits for testosterone levels.
- **Pumpkin Seeds, Red Meat, Oysters, Whole Grains, Seafood (Zinc):** These foods are rich in zinc, which is essential for testosterone production and maintaining a healthy endocrine system.

Incorporating these foods into a balanced diet alongside a healthy lifestyle will assist with optimising hormonal balance and overall wellbeing for men.

Male Adults (General) 7-Day Sample Meal Plan

	Day 1	Day 2	Day 3	Day 4	Day 5	Day 6	Day 7
Upon waking	Lemon juice or apple cider vinegar in warm water	Lemon juice or apple cider vinegar in warm water	Lemon juice or apple cider vinegar in warm water	Lemon juice or apple cider vinegar in warm water	Lemon juice or apple cider vinegar in warm water	Lemon juice or apple cider vinegar in warm water	Lemon juice or apple cider vinegar in warm water
Breakfast	Healthy Chocolate Protein Pancakes (p. 126)	Hot Smoked Trout & Pumpkin Breakfast Muffins (p. 136) V: tofu or omit salmon	Lemon & Coconut Buckwheat Porridge (p. 118)	Immune Supportive Manuka Smoothie (p. 110)	Zesty Trout, Walnut, Avocado & Lime Salsa Bruschetta (p. 144) V: tofu or chickpeas	Mocha Smoothie Bowl with Chai Spiced Nuts (p. 130)	Sri Lankan Scrambled Chia Eggs (p. 143)
Snack (optional)	Piece of fruit and unsweetened yoghurt	Piece of fruit and unsweetened yoghurt	Macadamia Hummus (p. 255) + veggie sticks	Roasted Beetroot & Hemp Seed Hummus (p. 250) on corn thins with avocado	Leftover Roasted Beetroot & Hemp Seed Hummus on corn thins with avocado	Leftover Pear, Banana & Blueberry Muffins	Unsweetened yoghurt with berries and nuts/seeds
Lunch	Egg Nutty Lunch Bowl with Creamy Avocado Dressing (p. 156)	Aromatic Indian Spinach & Coconut Soup (p. 152)	Leftover Aromatic Indian Spinach & Coconut Soup	Thai Salmon Salad (p. 194) V: tofu	Salad and avocado wrap with your protein of choice	Salad and avocado wrap with your protein of choice	Super Sausage & Mushroom Rolls (p. 192) + side salad
Snack (optional)	Macadamia Nut Pâté (p. 254) + veggie sticks	Leftover Macadamia Nut Pâté + veggie sticks	Piece of fruit and unsweetened yoghurt	Piece of fruit and raw unsalted nuts	Pear, Banana & Blueberry Muffins (p. 290)	Piece of fruit and unsweetened yoghurt	Leftover Pear, Banana & Blueberry Muffins
Dinner	Sumac Lamb Fillets with Cauliflower Tabouli & Coconut Tzatziki (p. 233) V: veggie patty	Chicken Thighs with Mushroom Sauce (p. 226) + steamed veggies and sweet potato V: tofu	Cashew-Crumbed Salmon with Lettuce Cups (p. 199) + optional steamed rice V: mushrooms	Eye Fillet with Nut Salsa Verde & Charred Green Beans (p. 216) V: veggie patty or tofu	Mini Spicy Chicken, Beetroot & Goat's Cheese Pizza (p. 214) v: omit chicken	Mushroom & Sweet Potato Shepherd's Pie (p. 228)	Warm Salmon & Zucchini Noodle Salad with Spicy Cashew Dressing (p. 205) V: tofu
Supper (optional)	Cacao Beet Brownies (p. 279)	Herbal tea and 2 squares of dark chocolate	Yoghurt with berries and nuts/seeds	Lemon Hemp Bliss Balls (p. 287)	Herbal tea and 2 squares of dark chocolate	Fruit with hemp seeds	Herbal tea and fruit

Case Study: Mature Male

John is a 32-year-old male who leads a physically active lifestyle, participating in daily exercise and running marathons. He recently got married and is looking forward to starting a family. While he is based in Australia, his job covers the American money markets, which often requires him to stay up late, affecting his sleep schedule. Despite this, his energy levels remain balanced, and he maintains a positive mood.

When John came to see me, his health goals were to understand metabolism, manage weight and stress, improve gut health, develop better eating habits and prepare for fatherhood. John has been diagnosed with irritable bowel syndrome (IBS), which contributes to his frequent flatulence and potentially impacts his overall gut health. His diet mainly consists of refined carbohydrates and eating out, which are not ideal for his IBS and overall health goals. His high-stress job, irregular sleep patterns and marathon training all contribute to increased stress levels, making his IBS symptoms worse.

Nutrition

To alleviate John's IBS symptoms, I asked him to limit certain carbohydrates that are hard to digest and can ferment in the colon, exacerbating gut issues. These carbohydrates are known as FODMAPs – fermentable oligosaccharides, disaccharides, monosaccharides and polyols – and are found in common foods such as wheat, onions, garlic, dairy products containing high amounts of lactose such as milk, yoghurt and soft cheese, fruits like apples and pears, and the sugar alcohols found in some artificial sweeteners and certain fruits and vegetables. I introduced prebiotic- and probiotic-rich foods, such as bone broth and miso soup, into his diet to support gut microbiome health. I educated John about the basics of metabolism and how physical activity, diet and sleep influence weight. When it came to eating, we talked about timing, portion control and ensuring all meals and snacks included lean protein, healthy fats, whole grains and a variety of fruits and vegetables. We also looked up healthier options for restaurants and takeaway in his area, so John didn't have to forgo eating out (which he likes to do).

In terms of supplements, John was using a whey protein powder that had a high sugar content. I swapped this for a minimally processed brown rice protein powder (containing fewer FODMAPs), and green powder containing coriander, wheat grass, aloe vera and milk thistle (to nourish his gut and liver). I also recommended he take ashwagandha, an adaptogenic herb, and magnesium to help with stress, mood and sleep.

Movement

Even though John is very consistent with his high-intensity exercise, he needed an activity that would help with his recovery and relaxation. He started incorporating yoga into his exercise schedule twice a week and discovered that not only did this help with his muscle recovery, but his stress levels also decreased and his sleep improved as a result.

Mind

John has incorporated a gratitude journal into his daily routine: on waking up each morning, he spends an extra five to ten minutes in bed writing down the top three things that he is grateful for in his life.

He has also started using the Insight Timer app, which provides him access to a library of free meditations and mindfulness exercises, which he has incorporated into his morning routine and even on his commute to work.

John is being more consistent with his going-to-bed and wake-up times, sticking to a similar sleep schedule on weekdays and weekends. He tracks his slumber hours using the Health app on his Apple iPhone and is working on his sleep hygiene: he now has a relaxing bedtime routine, playing calming music, turning the light down and avoiding screens for at least 90 minutes before bed. He also takes a magnesium supplement with ashwagandha, as they both have a calming effect on the nervous system and are slightly soporific.

Mantra – Find strength in vulnerability.

Connection

John has joined a yoga studio, where he goes for classes twice weekly. The studio is targeted at men and encourages them to take up yoga, which makes John feel more at ease than he otherwise would have in a typical yoga class, as they tend to be more female-focused. He has also joined a men's community group, When No One's Watching (WNOW), created by Tadhg Kennelly, a former Sydney Swans player, which has connected him with like-minded men with whom he gets along well.

Conventional Medicine

At my suggestion, John went to see his doctor to have his sperm count and quality checked, as fatherhood is a priority in his future. Results showed he was within a healthy range.

A healthy sperm count, also known as sperm concentration, is a critical factor in male fertility. It refers to the number of sperm present in one millilitre of semen. Typically, a normal sperm count is considered to be around 15 million to 200 million sperm per millilitre. However, it's important to note that fertility is influenced by various factors beyond sperm count, including sperm motility (the ability of sperm to move effectively), sperm morphology (the shape and structure of sperm) and overall semen volume. A comprehensive assessment of sperm health involves evaluating these factors collectively. Maintaining a healthy sperm count is essential for achieving successful fertilisation, but it's only one aspect of male fertility, and other parameters should also be considered when assessing overall reproductive potential.

John is feeling more knowledgeable about and in control of his diet and lifestyle choices. He continues to attend regular nutrition sessions with me, as he appreciates the support as he makes ongoing modifications to his diet to help his IBS, stress levels, sleep, marathon training needs and plans for fatherhood.

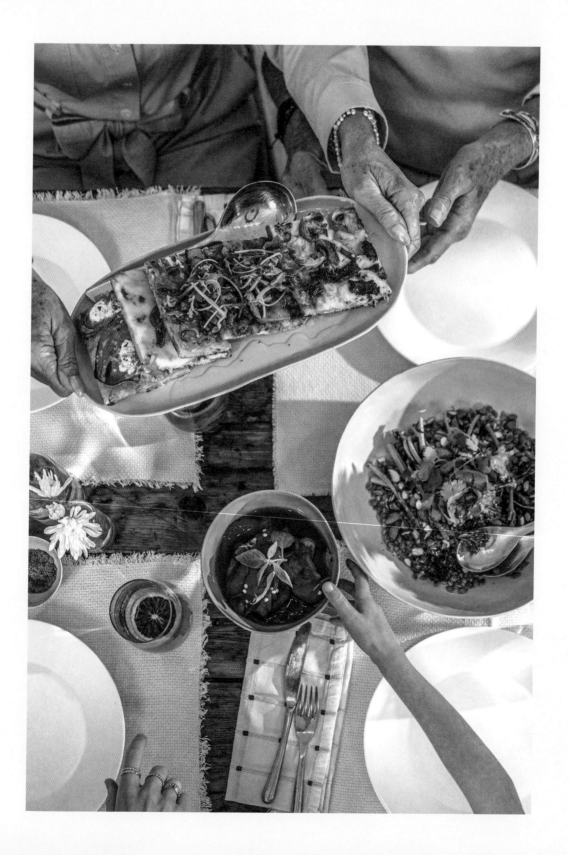

Recipes

Key

DF = dairy-free
GF = gluten-free
V = vegetarian
VG = vegan

Smoothies and Juices

DF, GF, V, VG • **Antioxidants**

Berry & Beetroot Smoothie

Serves 1–2
Prep: 5 minutes
Cook: n/a

1 small beetroot, peeled,
  grated/roughly diced/
  pre-cooked and diced

½ cup fresh/frozen berries

1 frozen banana, sliced

1 cup coconut milk/milk of
  your choice

1–2 tbsp yoghurt of your choice

1–2 tbsp raw honey, optional

mint leaves, optional

ice, optional

Place all of the ingredients into a food processor and blend
until smooth.

Pour into chilled glasses and enjoy.

—

*This family-friendly smoothie is a great way to hide veggies in
your kids' meals without them even noticing. Beetroot contains
betalains, which give beetroot its colour. They exert antioxidant
and anti-inflammatory actions in the body, making beetroot a
natural superfood. Kids often 'eat with their eyes', so they will
enjoy the colour of this smoothie.*

DF, GF, V, VG • **Healthy fats**

Brain-Boosting Smoothie

Serves 1–2
Prep: 5 minutes
Cook: n/a

1–2 cups almond milk/
  coconut water

1 tbsp almond butter

1 tsp virgin coconut oil

2 tbsp hemp seeds

½ cup frozen banana

½ cup frozen pineapple

Place all of the ingredients into a food processor and blend
until smooth. Add a little water to thin if needed.

Pour into chilled glasses and enjoy.

—

*For possible liver and antioxidant support, add ½ tsp fresh
turmeric.*

DF, GF, V, VG • **Magnesium**

Green Vanilla Smoothie

Serves 1
Prep: 5 minutes
Cook: n/a

30 g vanilla plant-based
   protein powder

½ tbsp MCT oil/extra-virgin
   olive oil

½ cup spinach leaves

½ cup avocado, skin and
   seed removed

¼ cup fresh/frozen blueberries

pinch stevia/raw honey,
   optional

1–2 cups water/milk of your
   choice

ice, optional

Combine all of the ingredients in a blender and blend until smooth.

Pour into a glass and serve immediately.

—

If you're having this smoothie around the time of a workout, swap the added oil for a handful of oats to help replenish glycogen and support healthy cortisol levels.

DF, GF, V, VG • **Antioxidants**

Antioxidant Matcha Cacao Smoothie

Serves 2
Prep: 5 minutes
Cook: n/a

2 cups milk of your choice

½ avocado, skin and seed removed

1 frozen banana, sliced

¼ cup fresh/frozen blueberries

1 handful spinach leaves

½–1 tbsp cacao powder

2 tsp matcha powder

raw honey, optional

Place all of the ingredients into a food processor and blend until smooth.

Pour into chilled glasses and enjoy.

—

Cacao and matcha are not only rich in antioxidants, but are also a source of magnesium, which may assist to reduce the release of stress hormones and positively impact our stress response. Magnesium is also a co-factor necessary to synthesise neurotransmitters such as serotonin and dopamine. This is the perfect smoothie to have to start your day with some mood-boosting ingredients.

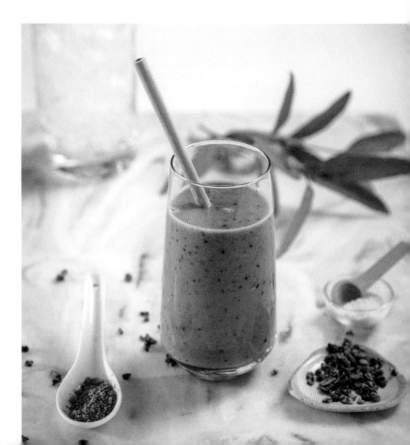

GF, V • **Vitamin C**

Immune Supportive Manuka Smoothie

Serves 1
Prep: 5 minutes
Cook: n/a

½ cup natural yoghurt

1 frozen banana, sliced

½ cup pineapple/mango, diced

½ tsp turmeric, grated/ground

2 tsp Manuka honey/
  good-quality raw honey

½ tbsp linseeds, sunflower
  seeds and almonds (LSA)

Place all of the ingredients into a food processor and blend until smooth. Add a little water to thin if needed.

Pour into chilled glasses and enjoy.

—

This smoothie is full of antioxidant-rich, immune-supportive ingredients. The bioactive compounds in honey may help to increase testosterone levels in males. For a dairy-free version, replace the yoghurt with coconut water or plant-based milk of your choice.

DF, GF • **Antioxidants**

Collagen Breakfast Smoothie

Serves 2
Prep: 5 minutes
Cook: n/a

2 cups coconut milk/milk of
  your choice

½ cup strawberries, chopped

½ cup banana, chopped

½ cup pineapple, chopped

1 tbsp chia seeds/hemp seeds

a few fresh mint leaves

2 tsp marine collagen powder

berries of your choice, to serve

Combine all of the ingredients in a blender and blend until smooth.

Pour into glasses and top with extra berries, chia seeds and mint.

—

If you're having this smoothie post-workout, double the collagen powder quantity to aid muscle recovery.

DF, GF, V, VG • **Antioxidants**

Watermelon, Strawberry & Beetroot Juice

Serves 2
Prep: 15 minutes
Cook: n/a

3 cups watermelon, seeds and rind removed

1 small beetroot, peeled

1 cup strawberry puree (blitz strawberries in food processor)

1–2 tbsp mint leaves, finely chopped

Juice watermelon and beetroot. Stir in strawberry puree and mint leaves.

—

Stir in 1 tbsp flaxseed or hemp seed oil as an easy way to boost healthy fat intake and support blood sugar regulation. This recipe is great for fussy eaters.

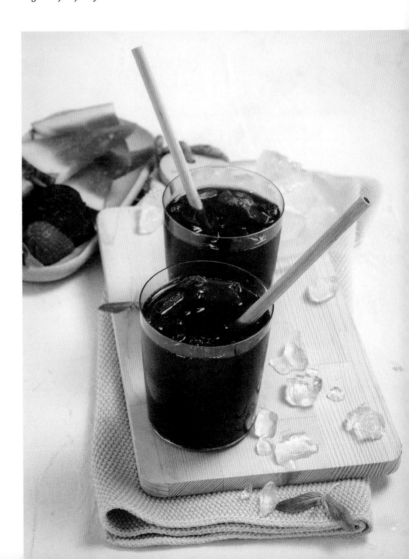

DF, V, VG   •   **Prebiotics**

Blueberry Smoothie with Avocado Mousse

Serves 1
Prep: 10 minutes
Cook: n/a

Smoothie

200 mL oat milk/coconut water

1 cup fresh/frozen blueberries

1 small frozen banana

½ tbsp whole rolled oats

1 handful fresh mint leaves

Avocado Mousse

½ small avocado, skin and
   seed removed

1–2 tbsp oat milk

½ tbsp lime juice

1 tsp maple syrup/honey,
   adjusted to taste

Topping

mixed nuts/seeds

mint leaves

To make the smoothie, add all of the ingredients to a blender and blend until smooth.

Pour into a tall glass and fill up 3 quarters of the way.

Add all of the avocado mousse ingredients into a blender and blend until smooth, then adjust the sweetness to your taste.

Spoon the avocado mousse onto the blueberry smoothie and sprinkle with the mixed nuts or seeds and mint leaves.

—

Blueberries contain bioactive compounds, including polyphenols and anthocyanins, which exert antioxidant properties that may help with cognitive decline and brain function. The addition of avocado to this smoothie adds an extra layer of support for brain health, due to its healthy monounsaturated fat content. This smoothie is the ideal breakfast tonic for those who experience brain fog in the morning.

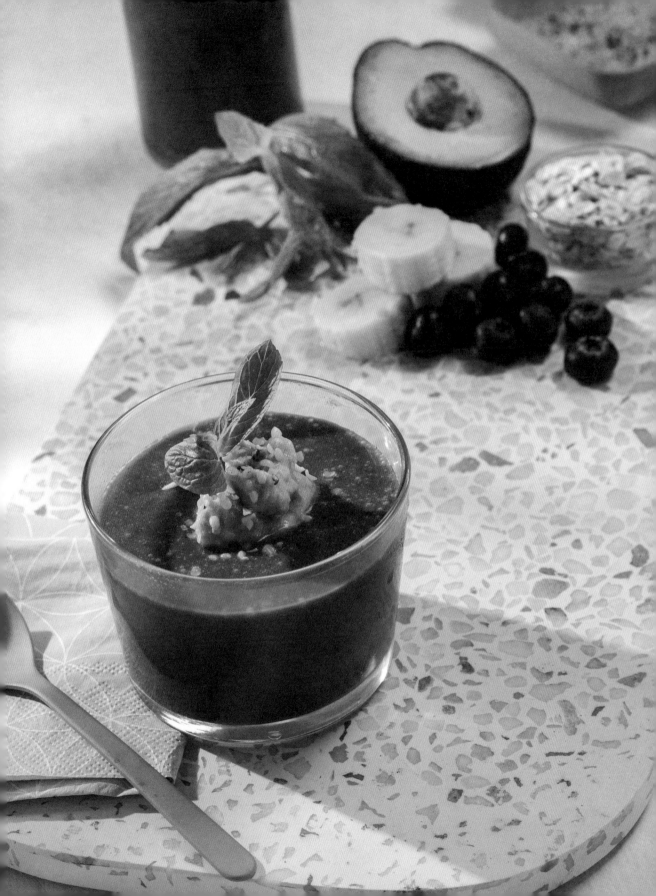

DF, GF, V, VG • **Antioxidants**

Green Matcha Frappé

Serves 2
Prep: 5 minutes
Cooking: n/a

1 cup coconut water

½ cup matcha tea/powder

1 cup kale leaves

½ cup mint leaves

½ cup cucumber, chopped

1 lime, peeled and chopped

½ cup ice, or more if desired

Place all of the ingredients into a food processor and blend until smooth.

Serve in a chilled glass with a squeeze of lime.

—

If you like to start your day with a fresh juice, this frappé is a great alternative.

DF, GF, V • **Vitamin C**

Kefir Turmeric Immune Tonic

Serves 1
Prep: 5 minutes
Cook: n/a

150 mL kefir/coconut water/
milk of your choice

¼ cup fresh pineapple, peeled
and chopped

½ tsp turmeric, ground/fresh

½ tsp ginger, ground/fresh

¼ tsp cinnamon, ground

1–2 tsp Manuka honey/raw
honey, to taste

1–2 tbsp extra-virgin olive oil/
virgin coconut oil

pinch black pepper

Add all of the ingredients into a high-speed blender and blend until smooth. Pour into a small glass, sprinkle with a pinch of cinnamon and enjoy!

—

Any leftovers can be frozen in ice trays. Add 1–2 cubes to your juice or smoothie.

DF, GF, V, VG • Antioxidants

Golden Coconut Milk

Serves 2
Prep: 5 minutes
Cook: 5 minutes

2 cups milk of your choice (e.g. coconut, cow's, almond etc)

1 tsp turmeric, grated/ground

1 tsp ginger, grated/ground

1 cinnamon stick

1–2 tsp honey, optional

pepper, to taste

2 tsp extra-virgin coconut oil

1 tbsp coconut chips, lightly toasted

Place milk in a small saucepan over a medium heat. Stir in turmeric and ginger until well mixed and drop in cinnamon stick. Continue to stir milk while warming through and add honey, pepper and virgin coconut oil.

Once warm, take off the heat and strain, then remove the cinnamon stick. Serve warm, topped with toasted coconut chips.

—

The active constituent in turmeric (called curcumin) is best absorbed alongside fat and black pepper, which is why coconut oil and pepper has been added to this recipe.

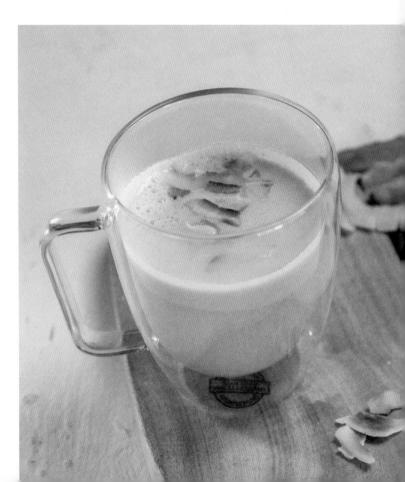

Breakfast

DF, GF, V, VG • **Antioxidants**

Acai & Berry Smoothie Bowl with Acai Choc Crumble

Serves 1
Prep: 15 minutes
Cook: n/a

Smoothie Bowl

2 tsp acai powder

1 frozen banana, chopped

½ cup frozen berries

½ cup coconut milk/milk of your choice

Acai Choc Crumble

¼ cup hemp seeds

3 fresh dates, seeds removed, chopped

1 tsp acai powder

1 tsp cacao powder

¼ cup walnuts, chopped

¼ cup macadamia nuts, roughly chopped

1–2 tbsp maple syrup + extra if needed

Other toppings

shredded coconut

fresh berries

goji berries

To make the smoothie bowl, combine all of the ingredients in a blender and blend until smooth (but still thick). Add additional milk if needed. Pour the smoothie mixture into a bowl.

To make the crumble, add hemp, dates, acai powder, cacao powder, walnuts and macadamia nuts to a food processor. Blitz the mixture using the pulsing function until roughly chopped. Slowly add maple syrup until the mixture starts to clump together.

Sprinkle the crumble lengthways down the smoothie bowl followed by a line of shredded coconut, berries and goji berries.

—

If having this smoothie post-workout, add some plant-based protein powder, as loss of oestrogen during perimenopause and menopause can make it harder to maintain and increase muscle mass.

Acai powder can be purchased in the health section of major supermarkets, at health food stores or chemists.

DF, GF, V, VG • **B vitamins**

Lemon & Coconut Buckwheat Porridge

Serves 1-2
Prep: 5 minutes + soaking
  overnight
Cook: 10–15 minutes

½ cup buckwheat, soaked
  overnight in 1 cup water
  then drained

1½ cups coconut milk/milk
  of your choice

2 tsp lemon zest

¼ cup shredded coconut
  (slightly toasted is lovely)

2 fresh dates, seeds removed,
  finely chopped

1 tbsp maple syrup/honey

1 tsp vanilla extract

fresh berries and hemp seeds,
  to serve

Add the buckwheat, milk, lemon zest, coconut, dates, maple syrup and vanilla extract into a small saucepan, bring to the boil and gently simmer with a lid on for 5–10 minutes until the buckwheat is tender and starting to absorb the milk.

Turn off the heat, keeping the lid on, and let steam for a further 5 minutes.

Remove the lid and fluff the mixture with a fork and spoon into serving bowls.

Top with the coconut, hemp seeds, berries and optional honey.

—

Buckwheat is a pseudo-grain and is a source of magnesium, which is considered a 'calming' mineral because it assists with regulating adrenaline and cortisol and helps your nervous system adapt to stress.

DF, V, VG • **Antioxidants**

Raw Fruit Breakfast Crumble

Serves 2
Prep: 5 minutes
Cook: n/a

Crumble

75 g whole rolled oats

50 g mixed seeds (hemp, chia,
   sunflower and pumpkin seeds)

50 g desiccated coconut

50 g fresh dates, seeds
   removed, roughly chopped

1 tbsp honey/maple syrup

1–2 tbsp orange juice, fresh

Fruit Mix

1 cup fruit of your choice (e.g.
   strawberries, pineapple,
   blueberries, raspberries,
   honey dew melon etc), sliced/
   cubed

½ cup natural full fat yoghurt of
   your choice

Add the oats, seeds, coconut and dates to a food processor
and roughly chop by pulsing. Add the honey or maple syrup
and continue to pulse until the mixture starts to clump
together, adding orange juice as needed.

In a small container or jar, place the fruit on the bottom, then
top with the yoghurt and crumble. Store the remaining crumble
in an airtight container in the fridge.

—

*This crumble is perfect for those mornings when you feel like
something different with a hint of sweetness, but you are short on
time. The fibre content of the oats and healthy fat content of the
seeds and coconut will leave you feeling satisfied, helping balance
the hormone insulin over the day.*

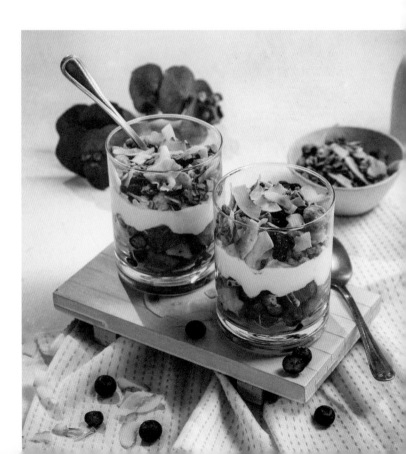

DF, GF, V, VG • **Fibre**

Fresh Coconut & Chia Bowl

Serves 2
Prep: 5 minutes
Cooking: 5–10 minutes

Chia Bowl

¼ cup chia seeds

2 tbsp fresh coconut,
shredded/dried

1–2 cups coconut milk

½–¾ cup fresh/frozen
blueberries

Topping

¼ cup nuts/seeds, crushed

½ banana/fruit of your choice,
thinly sliced

raw honey/maple syrup,
optional

In a small saucepan over a medium heat, place the chia seeds, coconut, coconut milk and blueberries. Cook for approximately 3–5 minutes or until chia seeds are translucent. Add a little water if you want to thin the consistency.

Serve in 2 bowls topped with the nuts or seeds and fruit of your choice. Add raw honey or maple syrup for extra sweetness.

—

This recipe can double as a calcium-rich snack, perfect for those avoiding or limiting dairy.

DF, GF • Vitamin C

Collagen & Acai Smoothie Bowl

Serves 2
Prep: 10 minutes
Cook: n/a

Smoothie Bowl

1 frozen banana, peeled and chopped

2 cups frozen strawberries/ mixed berries

4 tsp collagen protein powder

2 tsp acai powder/100 g acai pulp

½ cup coconut milk + extra if needed

Toppings

½ cup granola, gluten-free, optional

1 fresh banana, peeled and sliced into rounds

1 punnet fresh blueberries

⅓ cup shredded coconut

In a high-speed blender add all of the smoothie bowl ingredients and blend until smooth and thick, adding additional coconut milk if needed.

Take 2 jars, spoon a layer of the smoothie bowl into the base of each jar, top with a layer of granola, banana, blueberries and coconut. Repeat until all of the ingredients have been used. Finish off with a sprinkle of granola and coconut on top.

—

For added microbiome support, try adding a handful of oats (prebiotics) and powdered probiotics. Acai powder can be purchased in the health section of major supermarkets, at health food stores or chemists.

DF, GF, V • **Fibre**

Quinoa, Carrot, Zucchini & Apple Porridge

Serves 2–4
Prep: 10 minutes
Cook: 10 minutes

1 cup quinoa, cooked

1 small carrot, grated

1 small zucchini, grated,
   moisture squeezed out

1 small apple/pear, grated,
   moisture squeezed out

1 cup milk of your choice

1 tsp cinnamon, ground

1 tbsp raw honey, adjusted
   to taste

1 tbsp hemp seeds

Combine all of the ingredients in a saucepan over a low heat and let gently simmer until vegetables soften and mixture thickens, adding extra milk if necessary.

This porridge can be served warm or cool.

—

Quinoa is a delicious pseudo-grain which, as a 'carb', actually offers a good source of protein. The veggie addition means this porridge is also packed with fibre, which helps to regulate appetite and prevent snacking later into the day. To involve kids in this recipe, ask them to grate the fruit and veggies!

DF, GF, V, VG • **Antioxidants**

Turmeric Chia Berry Pudding

Serves 1–2
Prep: 5 minutes
Cook: 5–10 minutes

Pudding

¼ cup chia seeds

½ tsp turmeric, ground

1 tbsp vanilla plant-based
  protein powder

¼ tsp cinnamon, ground

250 mL organic coconut milk

1 tbsp raw honey/maple syrup

To Serve

¼ cup coconut yoghurt

¼ cup raspberries

2 tbsp macadamia nuts,
  chopped

In a small saucepan over a medium heat place the chia seeds, turmeric, protein powder, cinnamon, coconut milk and honey or maple syrup, combine well and stir regularly, for approximately 5 minutes. Add additional water to thin, if needed.

Once a pudding-like consistency has been reached, spoon into a bowl. Top with the yoghurt, berries and chopped macadamia nuts.

—

The active component in turmeric, 'curcumin', exerts anti-inflammatory and antioxidant actions in the body and helps to support detoxification and liver health. If you haven't tried turmeric before, this recipe is an ideal way to begin.

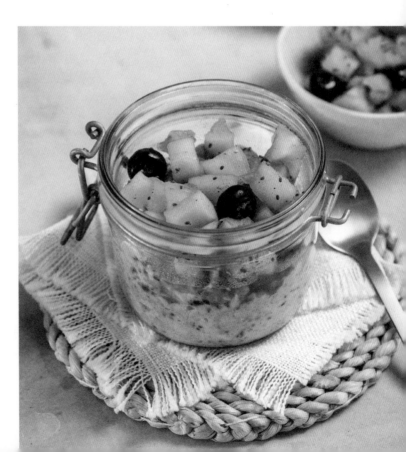

DF, GF • **Protein**

Bone Broth Chilli Scrambled Tofu with Roasted Smoked Paprika Tomatoes

Serves 2
Prep: 7 minutes
Cook: 20 minutes

½ punnet cherry tomatoes/
  1 vine-ripened tomato

1–2 tbsp extra-virgin olive oil

1 tsp smoked/regular paprika,
  ground

300 g hard tofu, crumbled

1 tbsp bone broth powder

1 red/green chilli, seeds
  removed, thinly sliced/
  ¼–½ tsp chilli flakes

¼ bunch parsley/coriander,
  chopped

sea salt and pepper, to taste

1 small Spanish onion, finely
  diced

1–2 garlic cloves, crushed

Preheat the oven to 180°C.

Place tomato on a lined baking tray, drizzle with the extra-virgin olive oil, and top with the sea salt and ½ teaspoon of paprika. Cook for approximately 10 minutes or until slightly golden brown.

In a bowl, mix together the tofu, bone broth, ½ teaspoon of paprika, chilli, parsley, sea salt and pepper.

Heat extra-virgin olive oil in a medium frying pan, add onion and garlic, and sauté for 5 minutes or until golden brown. Add the tofu mixture and gently mix for 5 minutes, until cooked to your liking.

Serve the tofu on a plate with the roasted tomatoes.

—

Eating adequate protein at breakfast is one of the most effective ways to prevent snacking and grazing late into the day. Adding bone broth powder to your eggs is an easy way to boost the protein content of your meals without much effort! Bone broth powder can be purchased in the health section of major supermarkets, at health food stores or chemists.

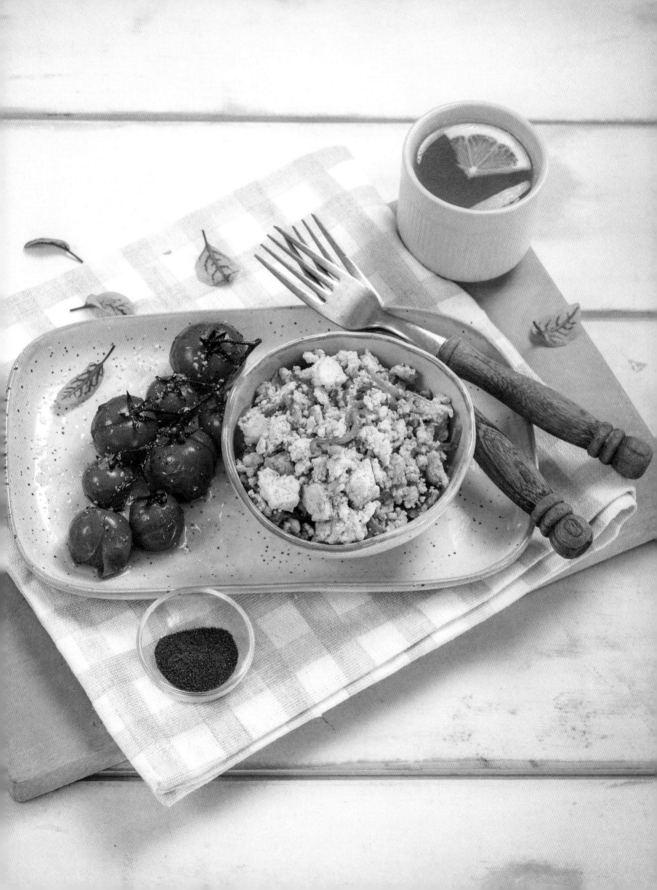

DF, V, VG • **Protein**

Healthy Chocolate Protein Pancakes

Serves 1
Prep: 10 minutes
Cook: 15 minutes

2 scoops chocolate plant-based protein powder

¼ cup LSA/hemp seeds

3 tbsp rolled oats

¼ cup natural peanut butter

¼ cup date puree/fresh dates, seeds removed

¾ cup milk of your choice/water

1 tbsp virgin coconut oil, melted/extra-virgin olive oil

a few squares of your favourite dark chocolate bar

banana/strawberries, sliced, to serve

Preheat a large non-stick frying pan.

Place all of the ingredients into a bowl and mix until just combined.

Lightly grease the pan with butter or cooking spray.

Cook large spoonfuls of batter until bubbles burst on the surface and edges start to go dry.

Turn and cook the other side until golden brown.

Serve topped with sliced banana or strawberries.

—

If you haven't tried LSA, it's a blend of linseeds, sunflower seeds and almonds! If not making your own, always purchase from the fridge section as this helps to preserve the oils from the nuts and seeds and prevent oxidation.

DF • Carbohydrates

Caramelised Pineapple & Coconut Butter Pancakes

Serves 2
Prep: 10 minutes
Cook: 15 minutes

extra-virgin olive oil/coconut oil, for cooking

1 cup pineapple, thinly sliced

2–3 tbsp maple syrup + extra to serve

1 cup self-raising wholemeal flour

1 tsp marine collagen powder, optional

2 tbsp coconut butter

1 medium egg

150 mL milk of your choice

shredded coconut

Preheat the oven to 180°C. In a hot ovenproof pan, heat the oil, then add the pineapple and maple syrup. In a large mixing bowl, add the flour and marine collagen powder. Add the coconut butter, egg and milk, and whisk until you have a smooth pouring consistency.

Pour the batter into the centre of the pan over the caramelised pineapple and swirl it to the sides of the pan in a thin layer. Place the pan into the oven for 15 minutes, or until cooked through. Flip the pancake onto a large plate, sprinkle with the shredded coconut and drizzle with a little extra maple syrup.

—

Pineapple is a good source of vitamin C, which is used by the adrenal glands to produce cortisol, our main stress hormone.

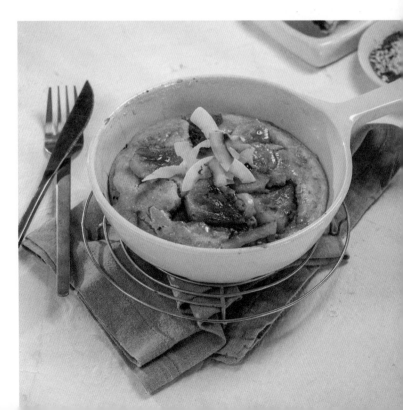

DF, GF • **Protein**

Miso Prawn Omelette with Tahini

Serves 2–4
Prep: 5 minutes
Cook: 10 minutes

Dressing

2 tbsp tahini

1 tbsp miso paste, gluten-free

water, to thin

Omelette

5 eggs, whisked

1–2 tsp miso paste, gluten-free

150 g raw prawn meat, roughly
  chopped

2 tbsp garlic chives, optional +
  reserve some to serve

1–2 tsp coconut oil, for cooking

Preheat the oven or grill to a medium-high heat.

To make the dressing, whisk the pastes in a small bowl or jar, and add enough water to create a pouring-like consistency. Set aside.

In a bowl, mix together all of the omelette ingredients, except the coconut oil. Heat a small ovenproof frying pan to a medium-high heat, melt the coconut oil and then pour the mixture into the pan. Cook for 3 minutes or until bubbling.

Place under the grill for 3 minutes or until lightly brown on top. Turn the omelette out onto a plate, or serve in the pan and drizzle with the dressing and a sprinkle of garlic chives.

—

For added fibre, chia seeds or leftover cooked brown rice or quinoa can be added to the omelette mix before cooking. Miso paste is available from the Asian section of major supermarkets, Asian grocery stores or health food stores.

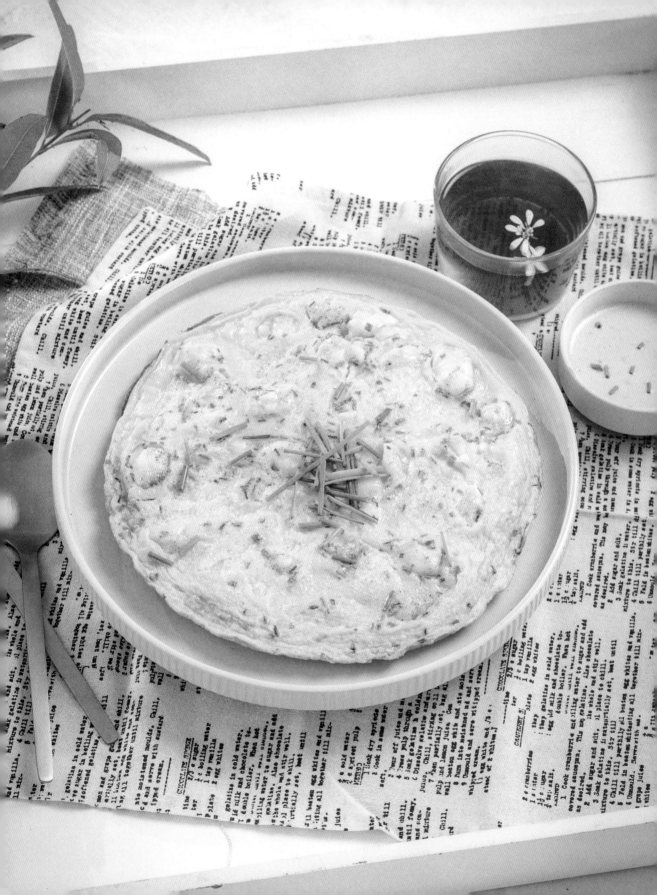

DF, GF, V, VG • **Healthy fats**

Mocha Smoothie Bowl with Chai Spiced Nuts

Serves 1–2
Prep: 10 minutes
Cook: 5 –10 minutes

Chai Spiced Nutty Topping

¼ tsp cardamon, ground

¼ tsp nutmeg, ground

¼ tsp cloves, ground

½ tsp cinnamon, ground

¼ tsp ginger, ground

50 g macadamia nuts

50 g walnuts

50 g hazelnuts

40 g extra-virgin olive oil

drizzle honey/maple syrup

Smoothie Bowl

2 tbsp chocolate plant-based
protein powder

1 tsp coffee beans, ground

125 mL water

¼ cup avocado, skin and seed
removed, diced

1 small frozen zucchini, cut into
chunks

handful ice

1 tbsp raw honey/maple syrup

To make the chai spiced nutty topping, preheat the oven to 180°C.

Add the spices, nuts, extra-virgin olive oil and honey or maple syrup to a bowl and mix well.

Pour mixture onto a lined baking tray and bake for 5 minutes or until lightly golden. Remove from the oven and let cool.

Leave chunky or add the nutty mixture to a food processor or blender and pulse until roughly chopped. Store in an airtight container.

To make the smoothie bowl, add all of the ingredients to a blender and blend until smooth. Add additional liquid if needed.

Pour into a bowl and top with 3 tablespoons of the nutty topping.

—

Zucchini instead of frozen fruit in a smoothie bowl may sound strange, but it actually adds a delicious, creamy texture! This is ideal for people who need to be mindful of their carbohydrate intake.

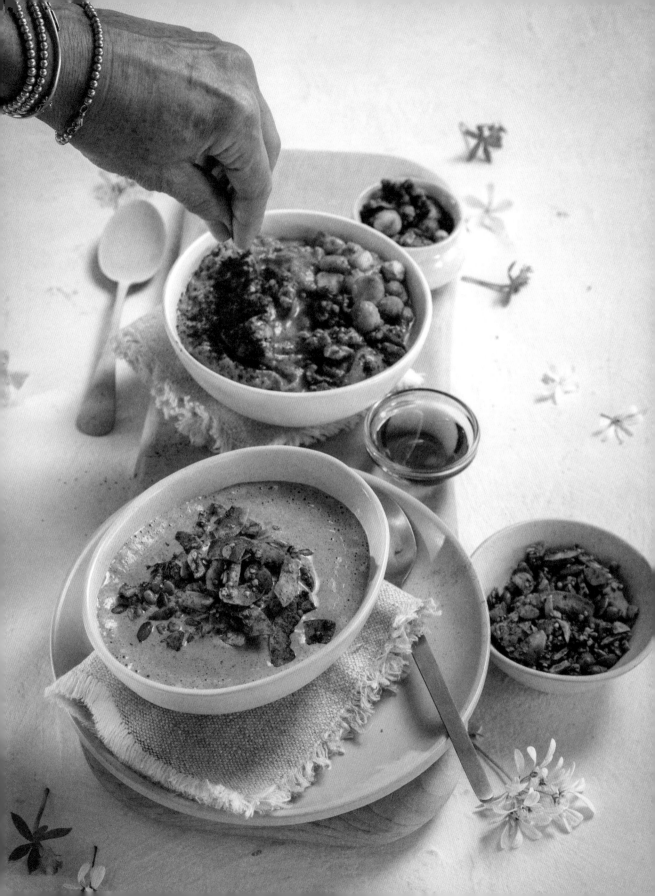

DF, V, VG • Complex carbohydrates

Golden Kiwi & Raspberry 'Cream' Oats

Serves 1
Prep: 15 minutes (+ overnight)
Cook: n/a

Oats

⅓ cup whole rolled oats

½ cup oat milk

2 tsp hemp seeds

1 date, finely chopped

pinch cinnamon, ground

pinch ginger, ground

Raspberry 'Cream'

100 g natural/coconut yoghurt

⅓ cup fresh/defrosted frozen
raspberries

1 tsp honey/maple syrup/fresh
orange juice

Toppings

½ tbsp mixed nuts/seeds

½ tbsp toasted coconut

1 golden/green kiwi, skin
removed, thinly sliced

2 pinches turmeric, ground

The night prior, in a tall jar, mix together oats, oat milk, hemp seeds, date, cinnamon and ginger. Store in the fridge with the lid on.

In the morning, mash together the yoghurt, raspberries and honey until well combined. If time permits, use a blender.

Remove the jar from the fridge and place half of the raspberry cream on top of the oats, then sprinkle with half of the nuts or seeds, coconut, half of the kiwi and turmeric. Repeat using the remaining ingredients.

Place the lid back on the jar and take it on the go.

—

Oats are a good source of B vitamins, which help the body to convert the food we eat into energy. B vitamins also support a healthy nervous system. Oats contain a good dose of soluble fibre, which helps with satiety and blood sugar regulation. This recipe is a good one for active kids to take on the go.

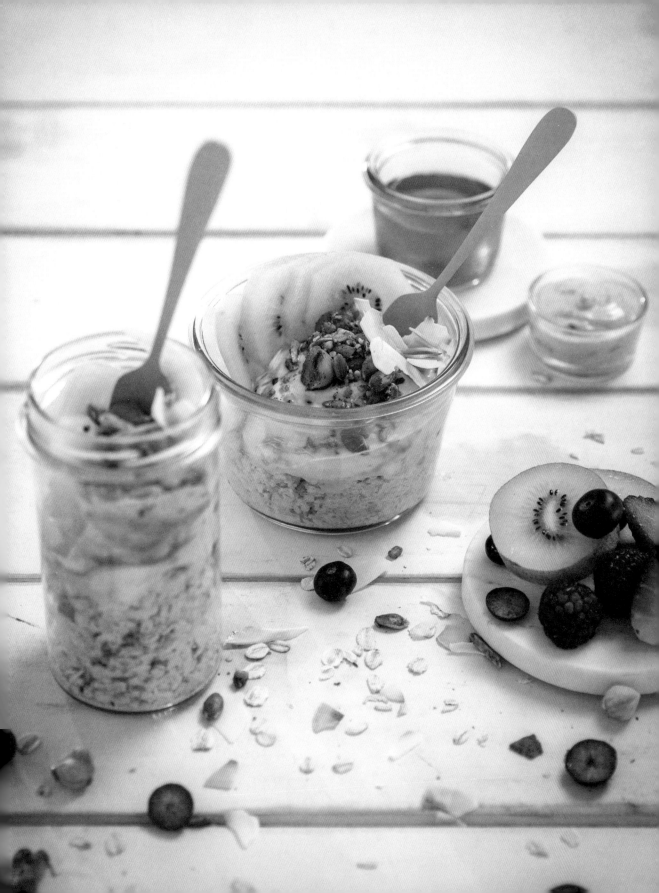

DF, V, VG • **Vitamin C**

Herbaceous Avocado & Roasted Capsicum Smash

Serves 2
Prep: 5 minutes
Cook: n/a

1 avocado, skin and seed
  removed, diced

½ cup capsicum, roasted, seeds
  removed

2 tbsp coriander, finely chopped

2 tbsp parsley, finely chopped

½ tsp lemon/lime zest

salt and pepper, to taste

1–2 slices sourdough,
  toasted/fresh

1 tbsp extra-virgin olive oil

In a bowl, mix together avocado, capsicum, coriander, parsley and zest, and season to taste.

Serve on sourdough, drizzled with extra-virgin olive oil.

—

Parsley, capsicum and lemon are good sources of vitamin C, which, when also paired with vitamin E–rich avocado, offers antioxidants that may help to reduce hot flashes.

DF, GF, V, VG • **Fibre**

Roasted Pear, Berries, Hemp & Coconut

Serves 4
Prep: 5 minutes
Cook: 20 minutes

Roasted Fruit

2 pears, whole

zest and juice of 1 orange

1 tsp cinnamon, ground

4 tbsp raw honey/maple syrup

2 tbsp virgin coconut oil/
   extra-virgin olive oil

1 punnet fresh blackberries

1 punnet fresh raspberries

To Serve

400 g natural Greek yoghurt/
   coconut yoghurt

4 tbsp flaxseed/hemp seeds,
   toasted

¼ cup coconut chips

Preheat the oven to 180°C.

Place the pears on a lined baking tray, drizzle with the orange zest, orange juice, cinnamon, honey and oil and bake for 15 minutes. Add berries to the tray, and bake for a further 5 minutes.

To serve, place fruit into 2 bowls and top each bowl with the yoghurt, seeds mix and a sprinkle of coconut chips.

—

Linseeds (flaxseeds) are not only a great source of fibre, but are also a phytoestrogen, which means linseeds may help to modulate the levels of oestrogen in the body. They are a helpful dietary tool for people with hormonal imbalances.

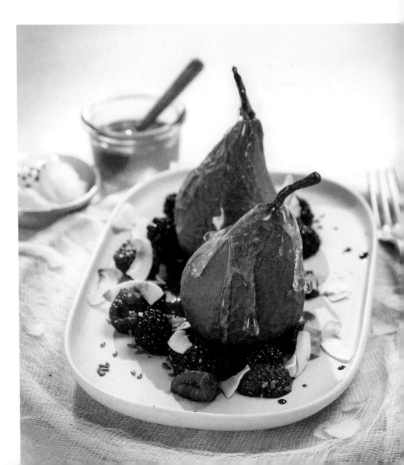

DF, GF • **Protein**

Hot Smoked Trout & Pumpkin Breakfast Muffins

Makes 6–8
Prep: 10 minutes
Cook: 45 minutes

1 cup pumpkin, peeled and diced into 2–3 cm cubes

1 tbsp extra-virgin olive oil + extra to drizzle

1 leek, outer leaves removed, finely sliced

1 garlic clove, crushed

1 cup kale, finely chopped

6 eggs, whisked

¼ cup milk of your choice

½ cup almond meal

200 g cooked hot smoked trout/salmon (you can use tinned/fresh salmon for kids)

½ cup cherry/grape tomatoes, halved

½ bunch dill/herb of your choice, finely chopped

toasted pepitas/pumpkin seeds

Preheat the oven to 180°C and place the pumpkin on a lined baking tray. Drizzle with the extra-virgin olive oil and roast for 20 minutes or until soft, then set aside to cool.

For the muffins, place a patty pan in each hole of a muffin tin. In a small saucepan, heat the extra-virgin olive oil, then cook the leek until translucent. Add the garlic and fry off for 1 minute. Add the kale and gently stir until wilted, then take off the heat and set aside.

In a bowl, whisk the eggs with the milk, then add the almond meal. Fold through the fish, cooked pumpkin, tomatoes, leek mixture and herbs and mix well. Pour the mixture equally between the patty pans and bake for 10 minutes or until set in the centre.

Once cooked and cooled, drizzle with more oil and finish with a sprinkle of the toasted pepitas.

—

These muffins are an ideal breakfast for kids and teens because they contain a good dose of protein to help stabilise blood sugar and energy levels up until morning tea time. Additionally, the omega-3 content of the salmon helps to promote brain function including focus and concentration. These muffins can also be taken on the go and eaten as a snack to fuel kids through sport and after-school activities.

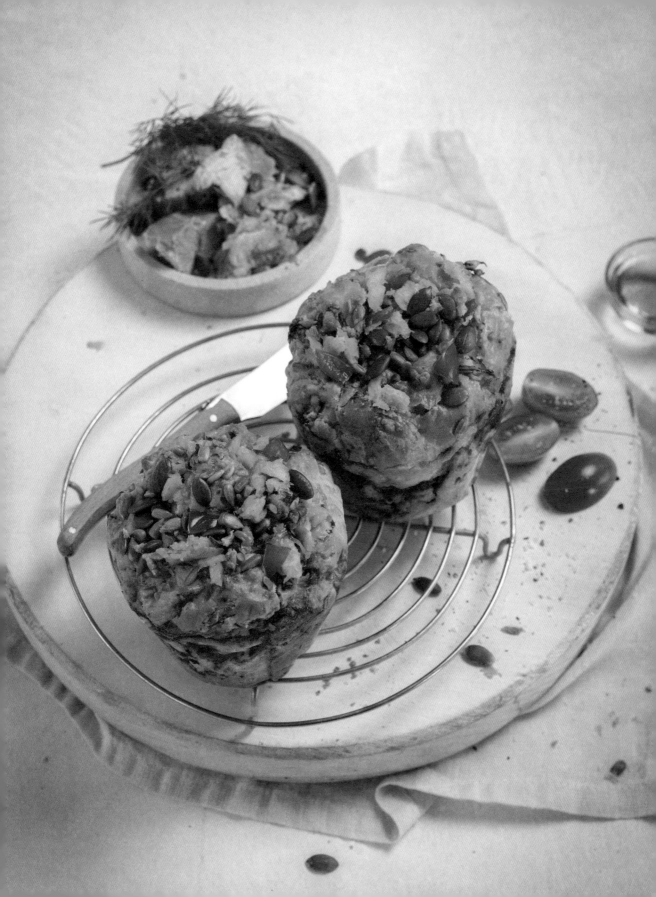

DF, GF, V, VG • **Healthy fats**

Blue Pea Breakfast Bowl with Maple Nut Granola

Serves 1
Prep: 10 minutes
Cook: 15 minutes

Maple Nut Granola

¼ cup slivered almonds

¼ cup macadamia nuts, finely chopped

¼ cup pumpkin seeds

¼ cup sunflower seeds

¼ cup flaked coconut

¼ cup hemp seeds

1 tsp cinnamon, ground

½ tsp nutmeg, ground

2–4 tbsp virgin coconut oil, melted + extra if needed

1 tbsp maple syrup

Breakfast Bowl

1 tsp blue pea powder

30 g vanilla plant-based protein powder

150 g natural/coconut yoghurt

½ cup frozen fruit of your choice

maple syrup, optional

fresh fruit of your choice, to serve

Preheat the oven to 150°C.

To make the granola, combine all of the dry ingredients in a bowl and mix well. In a small jug, whisk together the coconut oil and maple syrup, and combine with the dry mix, coating evenly.

Spread the mixture evenly over a tray lined with baking paper. Bake for 12–15 minutes until the texture is crunchy, making sure to toss every 5 minutes. Cool the granola mixture on the oven tray.

To make the breakfast bowl, add all of the ingredients into a blender and blend until smooth.

Pour into a bowl and top with the granola plus the fresh fruit on top.

Store the extra granola in an airtight container and refrigerate.

—

For a plant-based option use soy milk (made from whole soybeans) in place of yoghurt and increase the fruit quantity. Soy beans contain phytoestrogens. During perimenopause and menopause, consuming phytoestrogens may assist with symptom management. Blue pea powder can be purchased at health food stores or online.

DF, V, VG • **Fibre**

Vegan Apple & Cinnamon Nut Chia Oat Pudding

Serves 3–4
Prep: 5 minutes
Cook: 45 minutes

Compote

2 apples, peeled, cored and
  cut into small cubes

1 tsp cinnamon, ground

⅓ cup water + extra if needed

1 tbsp honey/pure maple syrup/
  brown rice syrup

pinch pure vanilla bean paste/
  essence

Pudding

1 cup whole rolled oats

3 tbsp chia seeds

2 cups plant-based milk of
  your choice

3 fresh dates, seeds removed,
  finely sliced

½ punnet fresh blueberries

⅓ cup mixed nuts and seeds

For the compote, place all of the ingredients in a small saucepan and cover with a lid. Cook over a low heat, stirring regularly, until the apple has completely broken down and the water has been absorbed. Taste for sweetness.

To make the pudding, combine oats in a saucepan with chia seeds, milk and dates. Simmer over a low heat, stirring constantly until the milk has been absorbed and the oats are cooked. Add extra milk if necessary.

Spoon into bowls. Top the pudding with a spoonful of the compote, blueberries and mixed nuts or seeds.

—

Adding chia seeds to your oats is an easy way to boost both the protein and healthy fat content of your meals. The compote doubles as a delicious dessert or snack – simply serve it with yoghurt and nuts or seeds.

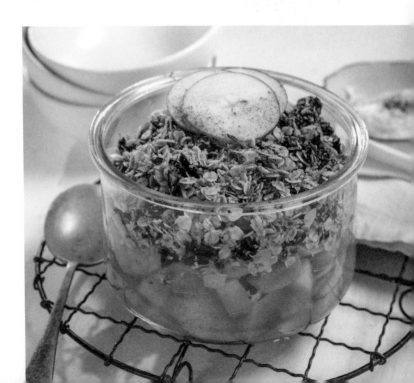

V • Iron

Savoury French Toast with Mushrooms, Goat's Cheese & Spirulina Pesto

Serves 2–4
Prep: 20 minutes
Cook: 10–15 minutes

Spirulina Pesto

1 bunch parsley, chopped

100 g walnuts

1–2 garlic cloves, crushed

½ cup fresh parmesan cheese, finely grated

juice of 1 lemon

1 tsp spirulina powder

¼–½ cup extra-virgin olive oil

pinch salt, to taste

French Toast

2 eggs, lightly beaten

¼ cup milk of your choice

sea salt and pepper

4 thick slices wholegrain sourdough bread, toasted

extra-virgin olive oil, for cooking

1 cup mushrooms, thinly sliced

¼ cup goat's cheese, crumbled

To make the pesto, combine all of the ingredients in a food processor and blend until smooth, then set aside.

Whisk together the eggs, milk, salt and pepper, then dip each slice of bread into the egg mixture and evenly coat. Heat the olive oil in a frying pan over a medium heat and cook the coated bread for 2 minutes on each side, or until golden. Transfer to a preheated oven to keep warm (optional).

Add more oil to the pan, then add the mushrooms and sauté for 4 minutes or until soft. Take off the heat and stir through half of the goat's cheese.

To serve, place 2 slices of toast on each plate, top with the mushrooms, drizzle with the pesto and crumble the remaining goat's cheese over each plate.

—

Spirulina contains large amounts of calcium, magnesium and potassium, which are important hormone-balancing minerals that can help reduce breast tenderness, inflammation and cramps. This savoury French toast is a delicious alternative to the sweet version. Leftover spirulina pesto can be used as a salad dressing (thin with water), sandwich spread, dip or added to omelettes and scrambled eggs. Spirulina can be purchased in the health section of major supermarkets, at health food stores or chemists.

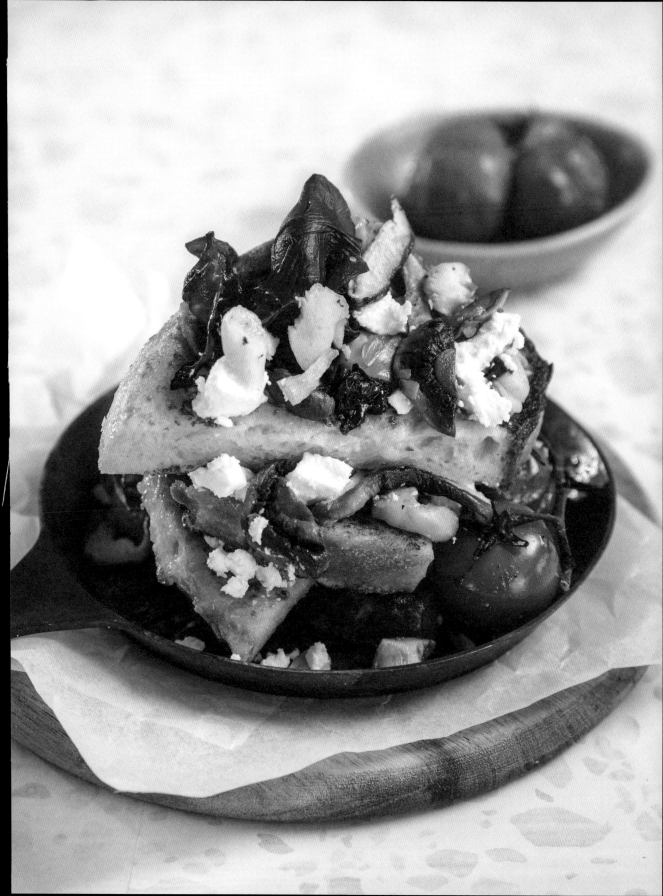

DF, GF, V • Selenium

Miso Mushroom Scrambled Eggs

Serves 2
Prep: 5 minutes
Cook: 5 minutes

4 eggs

1 tbsp miso paste, gluten-free, whisked with 1 tbsp water until liquid

2 tbsp extra-virgin olive oil

150 g mushroom, finely chopped

1 ripe avocado, skin and seed removed, diced

1 tbsp chives, chopped finely

salt and pepper, to taste

Crack eggs into a bowl and whisk before adding the miso paste mixture.

Heat extra-virgin olive oil over a medium heat, add mushroom, sauté for 2–5 minutes. Add egg mixture to the pan and gently scramble.

Before taking off the heat, fold through the diced avocado. Season to taste.

Remove from the heat and sprinkle with the chopped chives.

—

If you haven't tried miso paste, it is made from fermented soy beans and has a salty and umami taste. Miso contains isoflavones (a class of phytoestrogen) which have a similar structure to oestrogen. They may help with the symptoms of menopause, as they bind with oestrogen receptors. Remember, a little bit goes a long way and the lighter colour miso tends to have a milder taste. So if you're new to miso, it is best to start with a white miso paste. Miso paste is available from the Asian section of major supermarkets, Asian grocery stores or health food stores.

DF, GF, V • Iron

Sri Lankan Scrambled Chia Eggs

Serves 2–4
Prep: 5 minutes
Cook: 5 minutes

Coriander Sauce

1 bunch coriander leaves

1–2 garlic cloves, crushed

½ cup cashews

¼ cup extra-virgin olive oil

¼ tsp turmeric, fresh/ground

¼ tsp ginger, fresh/ground

juice of ½–1 lime

1 tsp lime zest

1 kaffir lime leaf

sea salt, to taste

water, to thin if needed

Scrambled Eggs

4 eggs

½ tbsp chia seeds

1 tbsp virgin coconut oil/
   extra-virgin olive oil

baby spinach leaves, to serve

To make the coriander sauce, blend all of the ingredients in a food processor until smooth, then set aside.

In a small bowl, whisk the eggs with 2 tablespoons of the coriander sauce and chia seeds.

Heat the oil in a pan over a medium heat. Add the egg mixture and gently scramble.

Serve the scrambled eggs on a bed of the baby spinach leaves with an extra drizzle of the coriander sauce and a sprinkle of the chia seeds.

—

Coriander has been traditionally used to support digestion and detoxification. This sauce can also be used as a salad dressing for added antioxidant support.

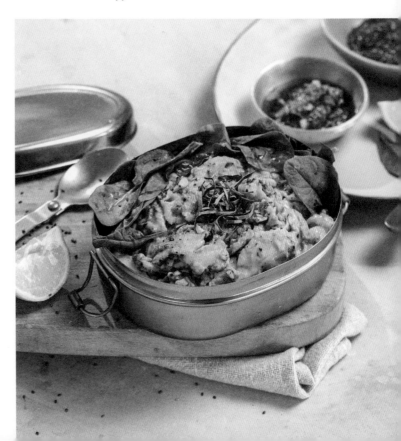

DF • **Healthy fats**

Zesty Trout, Walnut, Avocado & Lime Salsa Bruschetta

Serves 4
Prep: 15 minutes
Cook: n/a

100 g smoked trout, crumbled

1 cup walnuts, lightly toasted and chopped

1 avocado, skin and seed removed, finely diced

1–2 tbsp lime juice

2 tsp lime zest

½ punnet grape tomatoes, finely diced

½ bunch basil, finely chopped

1 green chilli, seeds removed, finely sliced

sea salt and pepper, to taste

4 slices sourdough bread

In a small bowl, combine trout, walnuts, avocado, lime juice, lime zest, tomatoes, basil and chilli. Mix well, season to taste.

Spoon the mixture on top of sliced bread.

—

Walnuts contain phytoestrogen, which can be beneficial in helping support healthy oestrogen levels.

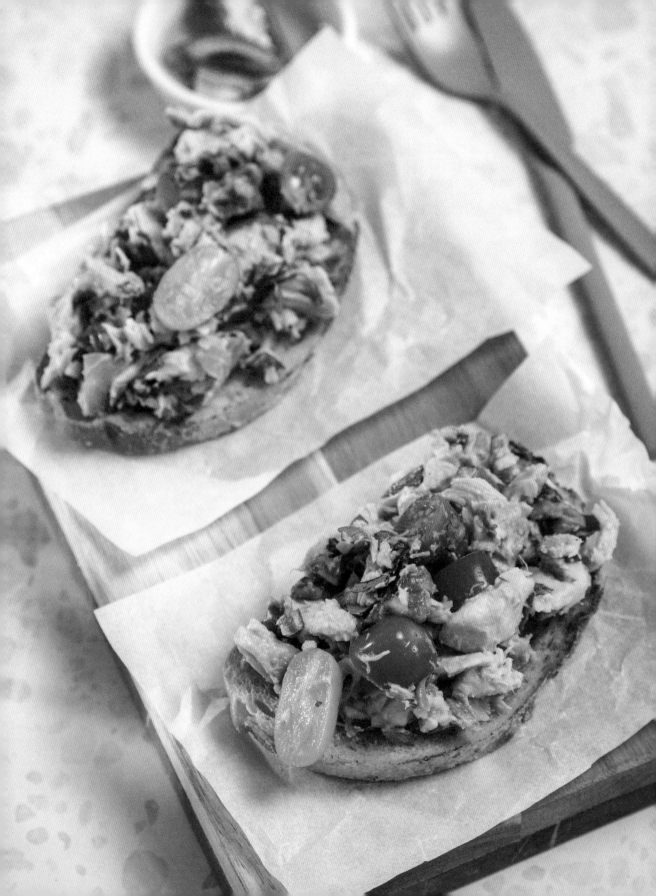

Lunch

GF, V • **Vitamin C**

Mushroom & Mozzarella Stacks with Pesto

Serves 2
Prep: 15 minutes
Cook: 40 minutes

Pesto

½ bunch basil leaves

1 garlic clove, crushed

25 g parmesan cheese

½ cup macadamia nuts, toasted

1 tbsp lemon juice

2 tbsp extra-virgin olive oil

Mushroom & Mozzarella Stacks

2 large Portobello/field mushrooms, stems removed

100 g pumpkin, skin on, cut into thick rounds

1 red onion, peeled, cut into thick rounds

1 large vine-ripened tomato, cut into 4 rounds

1½ tsp extra-virgin olive oil

100 g mozzarella cheese, cut into 6 slices

To make the pesto, combine all of the ingredients in a blender or food processor and blend until well combined. Add a dash of boiling water to thin if necessary, then set aside.

Preheat a griddle pan or barbecue to a medium-high heat. Brush the mushroom, pumpkin, onion and tomato with extra-virgin olive oil, place on the heat and cook on each side until tender and charred. Remove from the heat once cooked.

Place mushrooms on a plate, then layer with a slice of mozzarella, onion, another slice of mozzarella, pumpkin, 1 more slice of mozzarella, and finish with the rounds of tomato. Drizzle 1 tablespoon of pesto over the top of each stack.

—

If your liver needs extra support, try adding a few teaspoons of spirulina to the pesto before blending.

DF, GF, V, VG • Iron

Warm Roasted Vegetable Salad with Tahini Coriander Beetroot Dressing

Serves 4
Prep: 15 minutes
Cook: 25–35 minutes

Vegetable Salad

2–4 tbsp extra-virgin olive oil

12 brussels sprouts, halved

½ head cauliflower, cut into florets

1 small sweet potato, peeled and cut into medium pieces

salt and pepper, to taste

100 g baby spinach leaves

½ bunch coriander, leaves picked

1–2 tbsp flaked almonds

Creamy Beetroot Dressing

1 cup cooked beetroot

½ bunch coriander, roughly chopped

⅓ cup tahini

1–2 tbsp lemon juice

1 tsp lemon zest

1 tsp beetroot powder, optional

1 garlic clove, crushed

2–4 tbsp extra-virgin olive oil

water, to thin

Preheat the oven 180°C.

Toss vegetables in a baking tray with extra-virgin olive oil, salt and pepper, and roast for 25–35 minutes, turning occasionally until tender and golden brown.

To make the dressing, combine all of the ingredients in a food processor or blender and blend until smooth, adding water if necessary.

Place the spinach at the bottom of a bowl, top with the roasted vegetables, and drizzle with the creamy beetroot dressing. Top with the coriander and flaked almonds.

—

If you have trouble sleeping, swap cashews for almonds to increase the vitamin E content of this meal. Research has shown a protective effect of vitamin E on sleep quality.

GF, V • Vitamin C

Moroccan Carrot Salad with Garlic Citrus Aioli

Serves 4–6 (as a side)
Prep: 15 minutes
Cook: 30–40 minutes

Moroccan Roasted Carrots

500 g carrots, peeled and thickly sliced diagonally

3 tbsp extra-virgin olive oil

½ tbsp cumin, ground

½ tbsp coriander seeds, ground

pinch cinnamon, ground

½ tbsp pomegranate molasses

salt and pepper

Salad

100 g feta/goat's cheese, crumbled

½ cup fresh coriander leaves, chopped

¼ cup flaked almonds

Garlic Citrus Aioli

2 egg yolks, at room temperature

1–2 tbsp lemon juice/apple cider vinegar

1–2 garlic cloves, crushed

350 mL extra-virgin olive oil

Preheat the oven to 180°C.

Place the carrots in a baking dish, then drizzle with the extra-virgin olive oil. Sprinkle with the cumin, coriander seeds and cinnamon, and toss well.

Roast until tender and golden in colour. Once ready, remove from the oven then drizzle over the pomegranate molasses, salt and pepper and season and toss well. Place on a serving dish. Top with the cheese, coriander leaves and flaked almonds.

To make the aioli, blend the egg yolks, lemon juice and garlic until smooth by using a food processor or whisking by hand. With the motor running or while whisking, slowly add the extra-virgin olive oil until the mixture is emulsified. Serve drizzled over the carrot salad.

—

Liquid vitamin D3 oil can be added to the aioli before blending as an easy way to take your vitamin D3. Adequate vitamin D3 intake supports bone health during perimenopause, menopause and postmenopause. Pomegranate molasses is available from gourmet delis and some supermarkets.

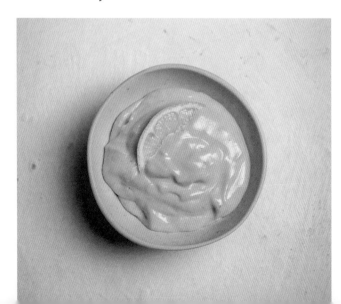

DF, GF, V, VG • **Magnesium**

Sweet Potato Noodle Salad with Creamy Cashew & Chia Seeds

Serves 2
Prep: 10 minutes
Cook: 20 minutes

Noodle Salad

250 g sweet potato noodle/ brown rice vermicelli/ konjac noodle

1½ cups rainbow slaw

1 punnet cherry tomatoes, halved

1 avocado, skin and seed removed, cubed

½ cup fresh coriander, finely chopped

1 tbsp chia seeds

Creamy Cashew Dressing

¼ cup raw cashews, roughly chopped

2–3 tbsp extra-virgin olive oil

1 tbsp tamari soy sauce, gluten-free

1 tbsp honey/maple syrup

juice of 1 lime

water, to thin if needed

Fill a large saucepan with water and bring to the boil. Add the noodles and cook for 10 minutes, to al dente. Leave to cool to room temperature.

In a blender, thoroughly combine cashews, extra-virgin olive oil, tamari soy sauce, honey, lime juice and enough water to make a runny consistency.

In a large mixing bowl, add the noodles and rainbow slaw, tomatoes and avocado, and gently combine. Mix through the cashew dressing.

Serve on a large decorative platter and garnish with coriander leaves and chia seeds.

—

Konjac noodles are made from konjac flour (an Asian root vegetable) and water. Konjac offers a source of fibre, while being almost devoid of carbohydrates. Konjac noodles are also very low in kilojoules and fat, which, combined with their fibre content, makes them a popular pick for weight management.

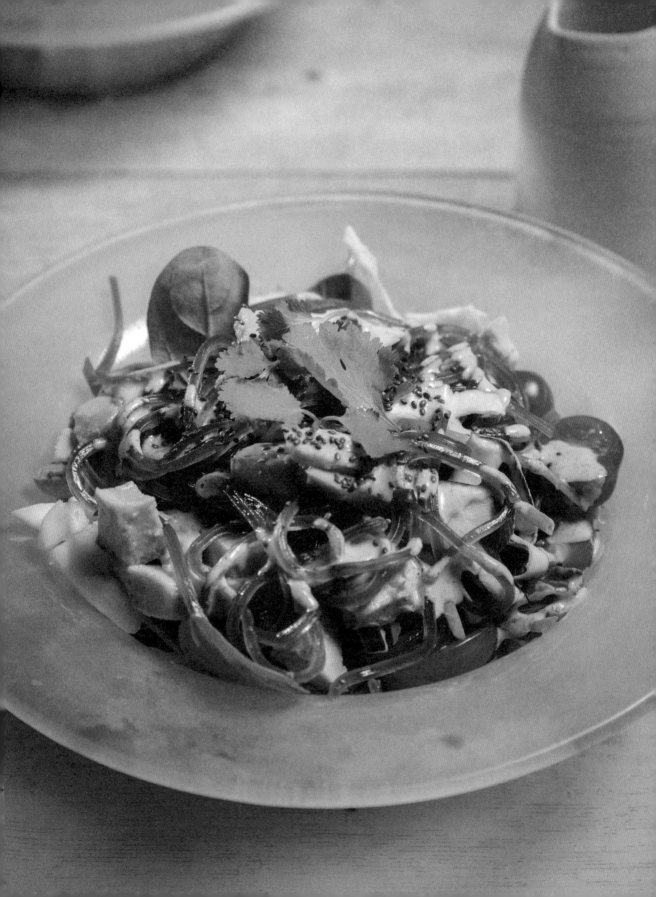

DF, GF, V, VG • **Magnesium**

Aromatic Indian Spinach & Coconut Soup

Serves 2–4
Prep: 15 minutes
Cook: 40 minutes

2–3 tbsp virgin coconut oil,
  for cooking

4 cups baby spinach leaves,
  roughly chopped

1 brown onion, finely chopped

2 garlic cloves, roughly chopped

½ tbsp cumin seeds

½ tbsp coriander seeds, ground

¼ tbsp fresh ginger, finely
  grated

1 long red chilli, seeds removed,
  finely chopped

1 L bone broth/vegetable broth,
  gluten-free

425 mL can organic coconut
  milk

½ bunch coriander, finely
  chopped

½–1 tsp sea salt, adjusted to
  taste

unsweetened coconut yoghurt,
  to serve

2–4 tbsp toasted sesame seeds,
  to serve

In a medium saucepan, add 1 tablespoon of coconut oil and sauté the spinach for a couple of minutes or until soft. Place in a bowl.

Add the onion to the remaining coconut oil and sauté until light brown, approximately 5 minutes. Add garlic, cumin, coriander seeds, ginger and chilli, and fry for a further 5 minutes.

Add the broth and coconut milk, then simmer for 10 minutes. Add half of the fresh coriander and sea salt, then stir through. Cool slightly, then blend with a stick blender until smooth.

Serve with a dollop of coconut yoghurt, sprinkled with the rest of the coriander and the sesame seeds.

—

Fresh turmeric also works well in this recipe in the same quantity as the ginger. Miso paste is available from the Asian section of major supermarkets, Asian grocery stores or health food stores.

DF, GF, V, VG • **Vitamin C**

Green Spirulina Winter Soup

Serves 6
Prep: 10 minutes
Cook: 30 minutes

2 tbsp extra-virgin olive oil

1 leek, outer leaves removed, finely sliced

1–2 garlic cloves, crushed

2 cups kale, finely chopped

1 head broccoli, stalks removed, roughly chopped

1 L vegetable stock, gluten-free

100 g raw macadamia nuts, roughly chopped

1 small bunch parsley, roughly chopped

2 tsp spirulina powder, optional

1 tbsp chia seeds, to serve

In a saucepan, heat the extra-virgin olive oil and add the leek. Cook until translucent before adding the garlic, then cook for 1 minute. Next add the kale and broccoli and sauté until the kale has wilted.

Add enough stock to cover the vegetables and bring to the boil. Simmer until the vegetables are tender, approximately 15–20 minutes. In the last 5 minutes of cooking, add the macadamia nuts, parsley and spirulina.

Take off the heat and blend until smooth using a stick blender.

Serve the soup in a bowl sprinkled with chia seeds and drizzled with extra-virgin olive oil.

—

To support healthy cortisol levels and to nourish the nervous system, stir through ½ cup cooked quinoa per serve after blending. Spirulina can be purchased in the health section of major supermarkets, at health food stores or chemists.

GF, V • **Protein**

Avocado Edamame Hummus

Serves 6
Prep: 5 minutes
Cook: n/a

1 medium avocado, skin and seed removed

½ cup chickpeas, drained

½ cup edamame beans, pod removed

½ cup zucchini, finely grated

1 tbsp Greek yoghurt

½ tsp raw honey/Manuka honey

1 tsp lime juice

In a high-speed blender, add all of the ingredients. Add additional Greek yoghurt to thin, or blend to desired consistency.

Spoon into a glass container and store in the fridge for up to 5 days.

—

Using edamame in hummus is a great way to boost the protein content of the hummus and this dish overall. This recipe makes for a yummy lunchbox addition.

V • **Fibre**

Avocado Edamame Hummus Quesadilla

Serves 1
Prep: 5 minutes
Cook: 7 minutes

extra-virgin olive oil, for cooking

1 wholemeal/corn tortilla or pita
  bread

2 tbsp avocado edamame
  hummus

2 tbsp carrot, grated

20 g cheese of your choice,
  grated

1 small handful spinach leaves,
  roughly chopped

Heat a little extra-virgin olive oil in a pan over a medium heat,
then add tortilla and spread with avocado edamame hummus.
Add carrot, cheese and spinach.

Fold in half and cook for 2 minutes or until lightly golden and
the cheese has started to melt.

Remove from the pan and cut into 4 triangles.

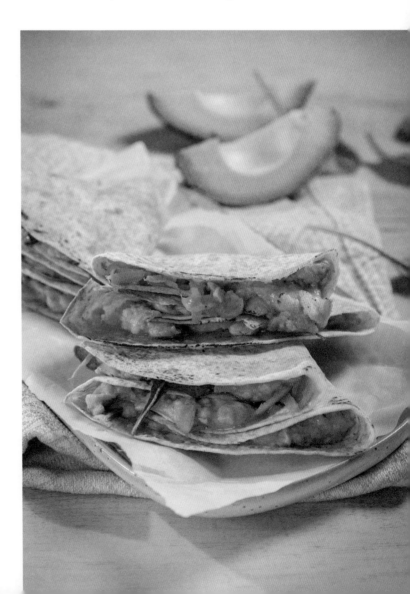

DF, GF, V, VG • Iron

Egg Nutty Lunch Bowl with Creamy Avocado Dressing

Serves 4
Prep: 15 minutes
Cook: 15 minutes

Dressing

1 avocado, skin and seed removed, diced

⅓–½ cup coconut milk

squeeze fresh lime juice

½ tbsp tamari soy sauce, gluten-free

1 garlic clove, crushed, optional

Toasted Nuts/Seeds

½ cup mixed nuts (e.g. cashews, walnuts, macadamia nuts etc)

1 tbsp pumpkin seeds

drizzle extra-virgin olive oil

pinch turmeric, ground

sea salt and pepper, to taste

Lunch Bowl

1 cup brown rice/quinoa, cooked

1 cup carrot, finely shaved/ grated

1 cup red cabbage, finely shaved

1 cup chickpeas, drained and rinsed

2 cups baby spinach leaves

½ cup cherry tomatoes, halved

4 eggs, boiled and halved (can use pan-fried tofu, cubed)

To make the dressing, combine all of the ingredients in a blender or food processor and blend until a dressing-like consistency is reached, adding additional coconut milk if needed.

For the toasted nuts, preheat the oven to 180°C and line a tray with baking paper. Combine oil, nuts, seeds and turmeric on the tray and mix well. Place in the oven for 10–15 minutes until lightly golden, tossing every 5 minutes. Season to taste.

In a bowl, mix the salad ingredients except the egg. To serve, place salad on a serving plate, and top with the egg, nuts and avocado dressing.

—

Sprinkle with chopped roasted seaweed for iodine to support thyroid health. Iodine is a mineral needed to help synthesise thyroid hormones.

GF, V • Complex carbohydrates

Beetroot & Goat's Cheese Risotto

Serves 4
Prep: 10 minutes
Cook: 30 minutes

extra-virgin olive oil, for cooking

1 leek, outer leaves removed,
　finely sliced

2 garlic cloves, crushed

1½ cups arborio/short grain
　brown rice

2 large beetroots, pre-cooked
　and diced

1 tbsp beetroot powder

3–4 cups vegetable stock,
　gluten-free

1 cup rocket leaves

200 g goat's cheese

salt and pepper, to taste

Heat the extra-virgin olive oil in a saucepan, then add the leek and cook for 4 minutes. Add the garlic and cook for a further minute.

Add the rice and stir for 1 minute, before adding the beetroots and beetroot powder.

Pour over 1 ladle of hot stock and continue to add stock at a simmer temperature, until the rice is tender.

Turn off the heat, stir through the rocket leaves and half of the goat's cheese. Season to taste.

Spoon into bowls and sprinkle with the remaining goat's cheese.

—

For a low-carb option that is still rich in fibre, replace the rice with 'cauliflower rice'. Beetroot powder can be purchased in the health section of major supermarkets, at health food stores or chemists.

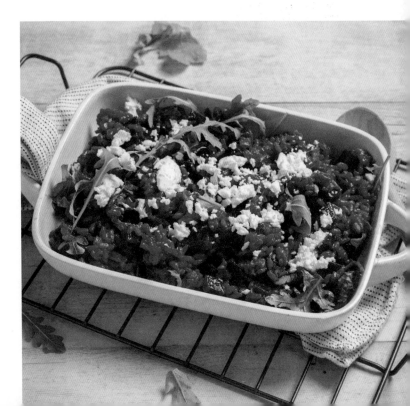

DF, GF, V, VG • **Selenium**

Broccolini, Brazil Nut & Quinoa Salad with Crispy Halloumi

Serves 2–4
Prep: 15 minutes
Cook: 40 minutes

Salad

1 cup broccolini, tips removed

1 cup cauliflower, cut into florets

pinch chilli flakes, optional

¼ tsp cumin, ground

¼ tsp sweet paprika, ground

salt and pepper

2 tbsp extra-virgin olive oil

2 garlic cloves, peeled

1 cup quinoa, cooked

½ cup coriander, roughly chopped

½ cup Brazil nuts, crushed

To Serve

1 tbsp extra-virgin olive oil

100–150 g halloumi/tofu, cubed

lemon juice, optional

salt and pepper, to taste

Preheat the oven to 180°C.

Line a baking tray with baking paper, then add the broccolini and cauliflower to the tray. Sprinkle with the chilli flakes, cumin, paprika, salt and pepper and drizzle with the extra-virgin olive oil, then mix.

Roast for 15 minutes, then add the garlic and roast for a further 15 minutes or until golden brown.

Once cooked, place the mixture into a bowl and toss with the quinoa, coriander and Brazil nuts.

Meanwhile, heat the extra-virgin olive oil in a frying pan, add the halloumi or tofu and cook until crispy.

Serve the salad in a bowl topped with the tofu or halloumi. Squeeze with a little optional lemon juice.

—

Using Brazil nuts in salads is a great way to boost your selenium intake. Selenium is a mineral needed for thyroid hormone conversion.

DF, V, VG • **Fibre**

Warm Charred Broccoli Salad with Herb Dressing

Serves 2 (as a side)
Prep: 5 minutes
Cook: 35 minutes

Dressing

½ bunch coriander, chopped

½ bunch basil leaves, chopped

1–2 garlic cloves, crushed

100 g cashews + extra to serve

juice of 1 lemon

2 tsp lemon zest

1 tsp sea salt, to taste

¼ cup extra-virgin olive oil

Broccoli Salad

½ cup pearl barley/freekeh/
  quinoa, raw

2 tbsp extra-virgin olive oil

1 bunch broccoli, cut into florets
  with stalks intact and halved
  lengthways

basil leaves, to serve

To make the herb dressing, blend all of the ingredients in a food processor until smooth, then set aside.

Place the grain in a saucepan with 1 cup of water. Bring to the boil and gently simmer for 20–25 minutes until tender (15–20 minutes if cooking quinoa), then drain.

Warm the extra-virgin olive oil on a chargrill or griddle pan and cook the broccoli on each side for 10–15 minutes until charred and lightly tender. If preferred, the broccoli can be roasted in the oven by laying flat on a baking tray drizzled with oil and baked for 15–30 minutes or until golden brown.

Combine the grain, broccoli and a few tablespoons of herb dressing. Top with the fresh basil leaves and a sprinkle of the extra crushed cashews.

—

This recipe can also be made with cauliflower in place of the broccoli. Like broccoli, cauliflower contains sulforaphane, a type of phytochemical which has potent antioxidant effects and may help to promote detoxification and liver health.

DF, GF   •   **B vitamins**

Pea Pesto Buckwheat Pasta Salad with Leftover Chicken

Serves 2
Prep: 10 minutes
Cook: 15 minutes

Pasta Salad

75 g buckwheat pasta/
   brown rice pasta

100 g leftover chicken/
   roast lamb, diced

8 cherry/pear tomatoes,
   halved

Pesto

2 cups frozen green peas,
   cooked and cooled

2 tbsp shaved parmesan
   cheese/nutritional yeast

½ bunch basil/spinach leaves,
   chopped

2–3 tbsp extra-virgin olive oil

½ garlic clove, crushed, optional

In a small saucepan, add the pasta and water and cook according to packet directions. Let cool.

In a food processor combine the peas, parmesan, basil or spinach and garlic. Blend and slowly add the extra-virgin olive oil until the mixture forms a smooth consistency.

In a bowl, combine the pasta and pesto, mixing well. Top with the meat and tomatoes.

Extra vegetables can be added, such as steamed broccoli, grilled zucchini, steamed carrot, capsicum, corn etc.

—

Using peas in this pesto adds not only a creamy texture, but also sneaks in extra fibre and protein! This recipe is a great way to sneak in extra veggies.

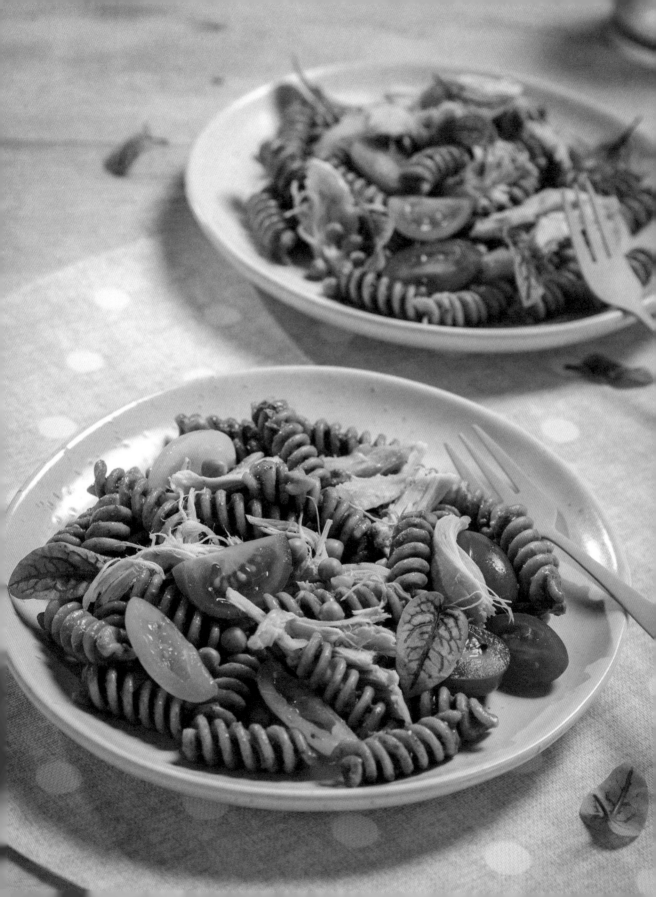

DF, GF, V • **Antioxidants**

Chia Beef Burger with Apple & Beetroot Relish

Serves 4–6
Prep: 15 minutes
Cook: 50 minutes

Apple and Beetroot Relish

1–2 tbsp extra-virgin olive oil

1 small red onion, peeled and finely sliced

1 tsp beetroot powder, optional

1 large beetroot, peeled and finely grated

1 green apple, cored, peeled and grated

2 tbsp apple cider vinegar

1–2 tsp raw honey

½ tsp cumin, ground

2 tsp sea salt

Burger Patties

1 tbsp extra-virgin olive oil, for cooking

500 g beef mince/hard tofu, crumbled

1 chia egg (1 tbsp chia seeds and 3 tbsp water mixed together and put aside for 5 minutes)

¼ bunch basil, finely chopped

½ tsp chilli flakes/1 red chilli, seeds removed, finely sliced

2 garlic cloves, crushed

½ bunch spring onions, finely chopped

2 tsp sea salt

2 tsp pepper, ground

chia seeds, for dusting

To Serve

4–6 wholemeal/sourdough seeded buns (or gluten-free buns)

1 tomato, sliced

1 avocado, sliced

1 handful rocket leaves

To make the apple and beetroot relish, heat the extra-virgin olive oil in a frying pan over a medium heat, add the onion and cook until soft, but do not brown. Add the remaining ingredients and let simmer for 15–20 minutes until soft and the mixture becomes sticky. Add a dash of water if necessary. Remove from heat and cool.

To make the patties, place all of the ingredients in a bowl and combine well. Shape into patties and sprinkle with the additional chia seeds.

Heat the oil in a frying pan and cook the patties on each side until cooked through.

To assemble, place a patty on a bun. Top with the relish, tomato, avocado and rocket leaves.

For a bunless version, serve a patty in an iceberg lettuce cup with toppings.

—

Pork in place of beef mince works really well in this dish and is also a good source of iron. Beetroot powder can be purchased in the health section of major supermarkets, at health food stores or chemists.

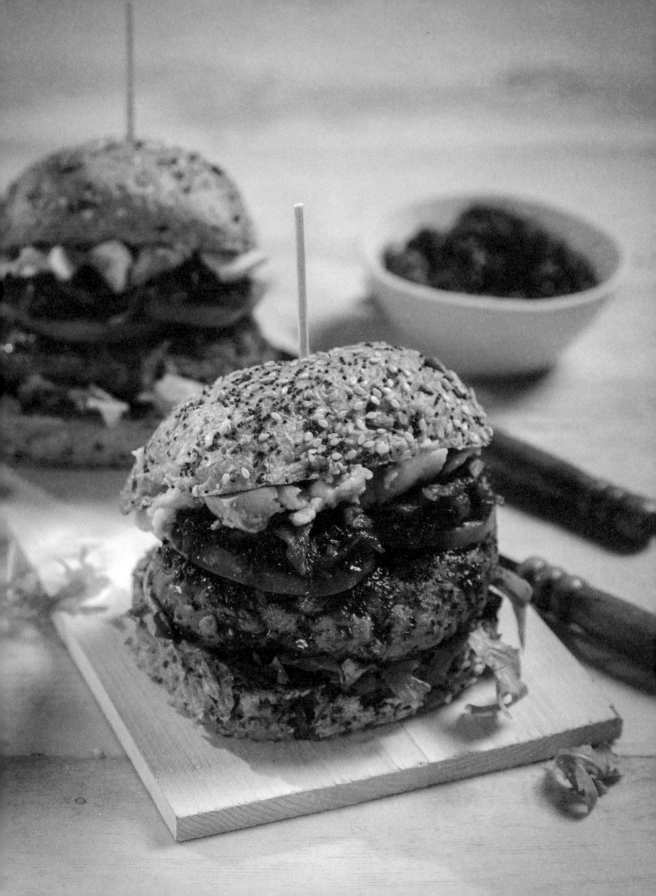

DF, GF, V, VG • **Antioxidants**

Fennel Detox Salad Bowl with Black Bean Hummus

Serves 2
Prep: 30 minutes
Cook: n/a

Black Bean Hummus

400 g can black beans, drained
   and rinsed

1–2 garlic cloves, crushed

⅓ cup black tahini/regular
   tahini

1 tbsp lemon juice

¼ tsp activated charcoal
   powder, optional

2–4 tbsp extra-virgin olive oil

sea salt and pepper, to taste

Salad

1 baby fennel bulb, outer casing
   removed, finely sliced

1 bunch watercress, stems cut
   short

¼ bunch fresh coriander, leaves
   picked

1 cucumber, shaved into ribbons

1 avocado, skin and seed
   removed, sliced

1–2 tbsp lemon juice

1 tbsp extra-virgin olive oil

2 tbsp flaked almonds, toasted

¼ cup pomegranate seeds

To make the hummus, combine the black beans, garlic, tahini, lemon and activated charcoal powder in a food processor. With the motor running, slowly add the extra-virgin olive oil until smooth. Season to taste.

To make the salad, gently combine all of the ingredients in a bowl, except the pomegranate seeds, and toss well.

To assemble the dish, place a smear of hummus on each plate and layer the salad over the smear. Sprinkle with the pomegranate seeds.

—

For added phytoestrogen support, sprinkle this salad with a few tablespoons of flaxseeds before serving.

GF, V • **Zinc**

Chickpea & Quinoa Greek Salad

Serves 2–4
Prep: 5 minutes
Cook: 20 minutes

Salad

½ cup quinoa, rinsed

1 cup water

1 handful baby spinach leaves

1 small cucumber, diced

8 cherry tomatoes, halved

8 olives, seeds removed, halved

2–4 tbsp feta, crumbled

1 tbsp pumpkin seeds, toasted

½ cup chickpeas/mixed beans, drained and rinsed

Dressing

1–2 tbsp apple cider vinegar/ lemon juice

1–2 tsp honey

2–4 tbsp extra-virgin olive oil

To cook the quinoa, place in a small saucepan with water and bring to the boil. Let it simmer for 10–15 minutes until water has been absorbed. Lightly fluff the quinoa with a fork and transfer to a bowl and cool.

In a small bowl, mix together all the dressing ingredients.

In a bowl, combine the quinoa, spinach leaves, cucumber, tomatoes, olives, feta cheese, chickpeas and pumpkin seeds. Add the dressing and mix well.

—

For extra creaminess and healthy fats, avocado makes a great addition – make sure to drizzle it with lemon to prevent browning. This recipe is a great way to introduce kids to salads.

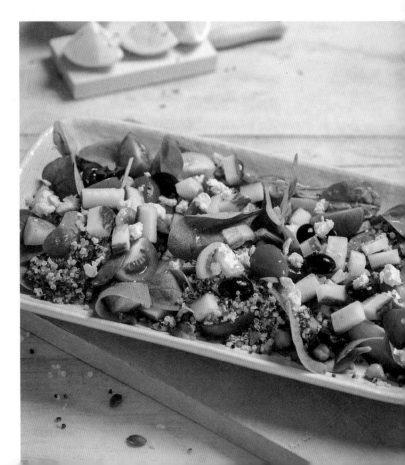

DF, GF • **Protein**

Chilli Seafood Skewers with Quick Asian Mayo

Serves 4–6
Prep: 30 minutes
Cook: 15 minutes

Skewers

300 g prawns, shelled and
   deveined

200 g scallops/firm fish,
   cubed

2 tbsp extra-virgin olive oil

4 garlic cloves, crushed

1 long red chilli, seeds removed,
   chopped into rounds + extra
   to serve

½ tsp Chinese five spice,
   gluten-free, ground

8–12 skewers

extra-virgin olive oil, for cooking

pinch salt and pepper

1 tbsp sesame seeds

Asian Mayo

½ cup egg mayo

¼ tsp sesame oil

1 garlic cloves, crushed

½ tsp ginger, freshly grated

½ tsp tamari soy sauce,
   gluten-free

chopped coriander, to serve

Soak wooden skewers prior to cooking.

In a bowl, add the prawns, scallops, extra-virgin olive oil, garlic, chilli and Chinese five spice, then mix well and let marinate in the fridge for 30 minutes (if time permits). Thread an even number of prawns, chilli and scallops on each skewer.

Heat the extra-virgin olive oil in a frying pan over a medium-high heat. Add skewers and cook on each side for a few minutes until cooked through. Repeat with remaining skewers.

Place on a serving plate and sprinkle with salt, pepper, sesame seeds and chopped chilli.

To make the mayo, mix all of the ingredients in a bowl.

Serve the mayo alongside the skewers and sprinkle with the coriander.

—

If you aren't a chilli fan, omit and replace with fresh ginger.

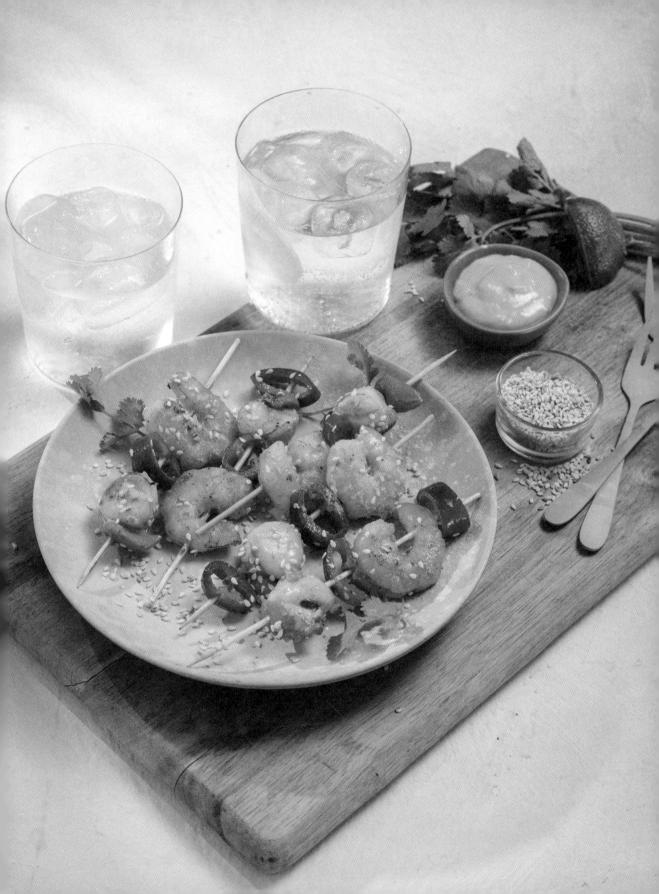

DF, GF • **Healthy fats**

Chilli & Nut Crusted Baked Fish with Cabbage Mint Salad

Serves 2
Prep: 20 minutes
Cook: 15 minutes

Baked Fish

1 tbsp macadamia nuts

½ tsp red chilli flakes

½ tbsp shredded coconut

1 tbsp hemp seeds

1–2 tsp lemon zest

sea salt and pepper, to taste

2 tbsp coriander, finely chopped

2 × 100–150 g fillets
   barramundi/other white fish

1–2 tbsp extra-virgin olive oil

Salad

1 cup cabbage, shredded

½ cup mint, optional

½ avocado, cubed

2 tbsp extra-virgin olive oil

1 tbsp apple cider vinegar

Preheat the oven to 180°C. Line a baking tray with baking paper.

Place the macadamia nuts in a food processor and pulse until a breadcrumb-like consistency starts to form.

Pour into a mixing bowl, add the chilli flakes, coconut, hemp seeds, lemon zest, salt, pepper and coriander, and mix well.

Divide the nut topping among the fish fillets and press down, coating evenly. Drizzle fillets with extra-virgin olive oil and place in the oven for 15 minutes or until cooked through and the top starts to look golden.

Meanwhile, add the salad ingredients to a bowl and gently mix.

Serve the salad arranged on a plate, topped with the fish. Drizzle a little extra-virgin olive oil on top.

—

If having spicy foods for dinner affects your sleep, omit the chilli and replace it with smoked paprika (mild).

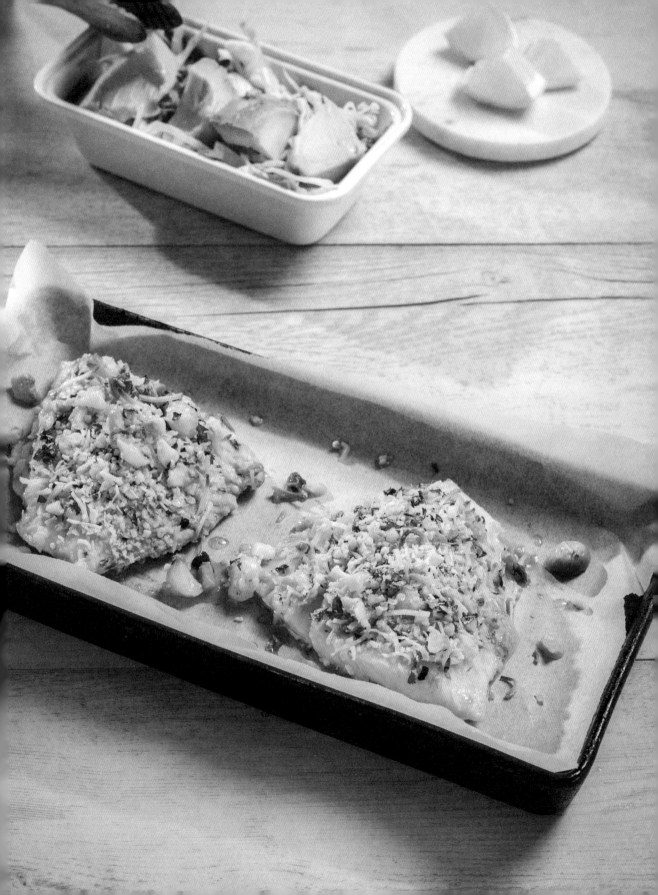

GF, V • **Protein**

Leek, Macadamia & Turmeric Frittatas

Serves 12
Prep: 10 minutes
Cook: 40 minutes

25 mL extra-virgin olive oil
  + 5 mL for cooking

1 leek, outer leaves removed,
  finely sliced

2 garlic cloves, crushed

2 cups kale leaves, roughly
  chopped

8 eggs

1–2 tsp turmeric, ground

sea salt and pepper,
  to taste

150 g fresh ricotta cheese

100 g feta, crumbled

½ bunch parsley, finely
  chopped

100 g macadamia nuts,
  chopped

Preheat the oven to 180°C.

Place 12 muffin patty pan cases into a muffin tin.

Heat 5 mL extra-virgin olive oil in a frying pan, then add the leek and cook for 3 minutes or until starting to slightly colour. Add the garlic and cook for a further minute. Add the kale leaves and sauté until wilted, then remove from the heat and let cool slightly.

In a large mixing bowl, whisk the eggs, turmeric, extra-virgin olive oil, salt and pepper until well combined. Add the ricotta, feta, parsley and kale mixture, and stir well.

Spoon the mixture into individual patty pans and sprinkle the tops with the macadamia nuts.

Cook in the oven for 20–25 minutes or until set and slightly golden on top.

—

For a nut-free version, which is still rich in healthy fats, swap macadamia nuts for hemp seeds!

DF, GF, V • **Antioxidants**

Finger Eggplant, Herb, Pepita & Pomegranate Salad

Serves 4
Prep: 15 minutes
Cook: 20 minutes

Salad

8 finger eggplants, tops removed, halved lengthways

1 tbsp extra-virgin olive oil

½ cup roasted pepitas/pumpkin seeds

1 bunch coriander, stems removed, chopped

1 bunch parsley, stems removed, chopped

seeds from 1 pomegranate

Dressing

2 tbsp extra-virgin olive oil

1 tbsp pomegranate molasses

1 tbsp lemon juice

1 tsp honey

½ tsp cumin, ground

salt and pepper, to taste

Preheat the oven to 180°C.

Line a baking tray with baking paper. Toss the finger eggplants in extra-virgin olive oil and spread evenly on the baking tray. Roast in the oven for 15–20 minutes until nicely roasted and soft to touch. Set aside to cool.

In a large bowl, add the roasted finger eggplants, pepitas, coriander, parsley and pomegranate seeds, and toss well.

In a small bowl, mix together the dressing ingredients.

Pour the dressing over the salad and mix well. Serve immediately or set aside in the fridge.

—

Pomegranate juice has been shown to increase testosterone levels in both men and women. Pomegranates contain punicalagins, which exert potent antioxidant properties. Pomegranate molasses is available from gourmet delis and some supermarkets.

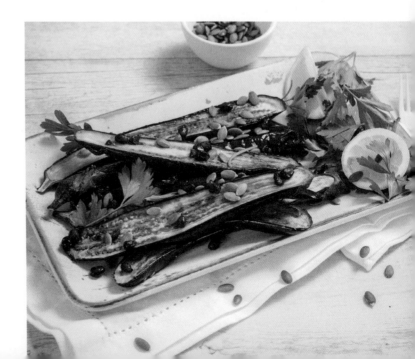

DF, GF • **Vitamin C**

Fragrant Chicken or Tofu Larb Salad with Turmeric Cauliflower Rice

Serves 2
Prep: 30 minutes
Cook: 20 minutes

Cauliflower Rice

1 small head cauliflower

1 tbsp extra-virgin olive oil

1 tsp turmeric, ground

¼ tsp pepper, ground

1 tsp sea salt, to taste

Larb

1 tbsp extra-virgin olive oil,
    for cooking

1 shallot, finely chopped

1 garlic clove, chopped

1 stalk lemongrass, bashed and
    finely chopped

1 tbsp fresh ginger, finely grated

1 red chilli, seeds removed,
    thinly sliced + extra to serve

200 g chicken mince/hard tofu,
    crumbled

¼ bunch mint leaves

¼ bunch coriander leaves

1–2 tbsp fish sauce, gluten-free
    + extra to serve

2 tbsp lime juice

lime, quartered, to serve

¼ cup shredded coconut

To make the cauliflower rice, add the florets of cauliflower into a food processor and pulse until the cauliflower resembles rice grains. Repeat until all of the cauliflower has been used.

Heat the extra-virgin olive oil in a frying pan. Add the turmeric and pepper and fry off for 1 minute before adding the cauliflower rice. Stir-fry for 3 minutes or until golden in colour and tender. Season with salt and set aside.

To make the larb, heat the extra-virgin olive oil in a frying pan, then add the shallots and cook for 3 minutes. Add the garlic, lemongrass, ginger and chilli, then cook for a further minute. Add the mince or tofu to the pan and cook for 3 minutes or until well browned.

Add half of the herbs, fish sauce and lime juice, and stir-fry for 1 minute until well combined, then adjust seasoning to suit.

Spoon the cauliflower rice into a bowl, top with the larb and finish with the extra herbs, coconut, freshly sliced chilli and a wedge of lime.

—

For active people who respond better to including complex carbs at each meal, use half brown rice and half cauliflower rice.

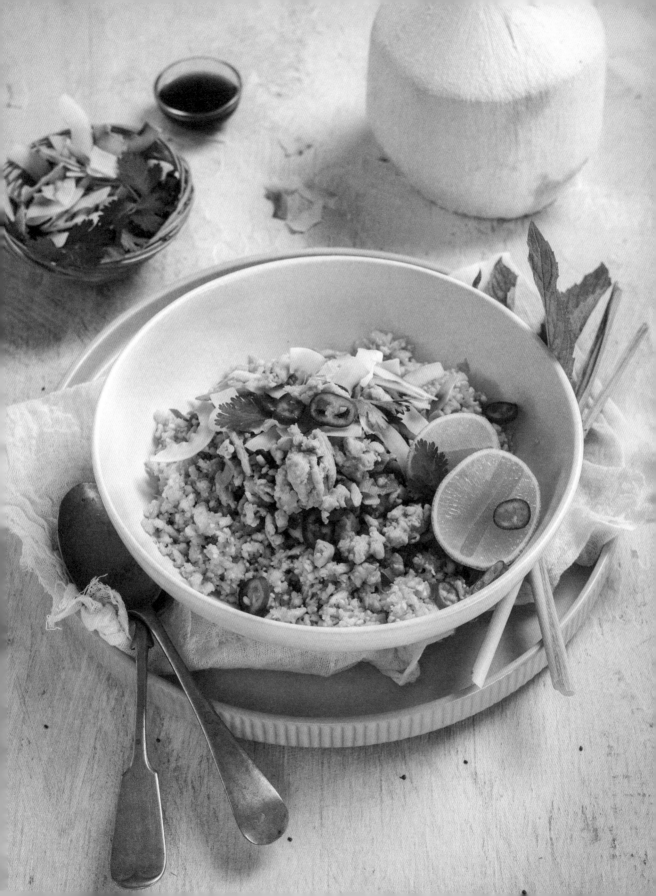

DF, GF • **Protein**

Garlic Prawns with Orange Zest Aioli

Serves 2–4
Prep: 15 minutes (+ 30 minutes
  marinating time)
Cook: 20 minutes

Prawns

500 g prawns, shelled and
  deveined

2 tbsp extra-virgin olive oil
  + extra for cooking

1 tbsp orange zest

1 red chilli, seeds removed,
  finely sliced, optional + extra
  to serve

pinch salt and pepper

chives, finely chopped, to serve

4 garlic cloves, thinly sliced

Orange Zest Aioli

2 egg yolks, at room
  temperature

1–2 tbsp lemon juice/orange
  juice/apple cider vinegar

1 tsp orange zest

1–2 garlic cloves, crushed

350 mL extra-virgin olive oil

To Serve

chives, finely chopped

rocket/baby spinach

avocado, skin and seed
  removed, diced

drizzle extra-virgin olive oil

In a bowl, add the prawns, extra-virgin olive oil, orange zest
and chilli, mix well and let marinate in the fridge for 30 minutes
(if time permits).

Heat the extra-virgin olive oil in a frying pan over a medium-
high heat and add the marinated prawns in small batches.
Cook on each side for a few minutes until cooked through,
then repeat with the remaining prawns. Once cooked, sprinkle
with the salt, pepper, chilli and chives.

On a high heat add the extra-virgin olive oil and fry the garlic
slices until golden brown, approximately 1–2 minutes.

To make the aioli, blend the egg yolks, juice, orange zest and
garlic until smooth by using a food processor or whisking by
hand. With the motor running or while whisking, slowly add the
extra-virgin olive oil until the mixture is emulsified.

Serve the aioli alongside the prawns and sprinkle the fried
garlic on top. Serve with the chives, rocket or baby spinach,
avocado and a drizzle of extra-virgin olive oil.

—

If you aren't a fan of prawns, the marinade works well with
scallops, calamari, fish and even chicken.

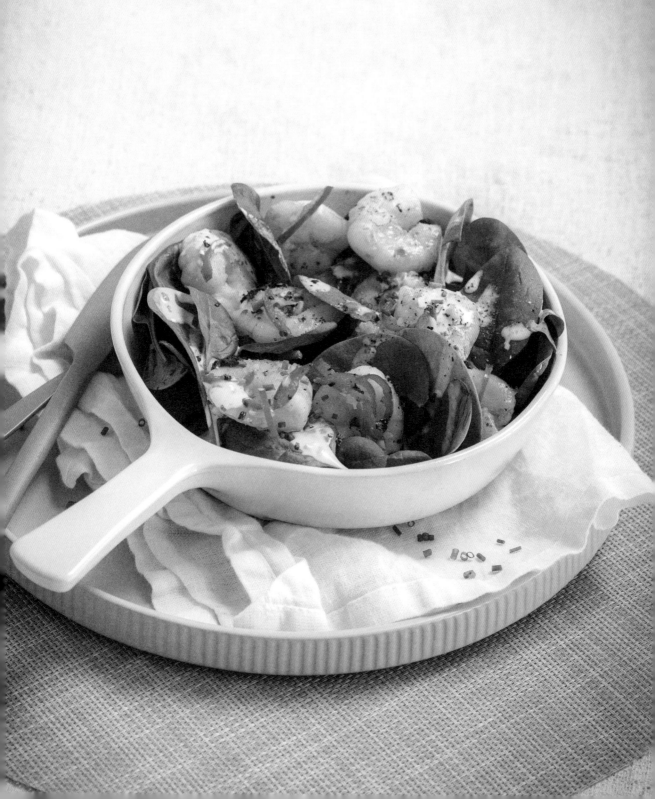

DF, V, VG   •   **Selenium**

Ginger Miso Tofu Nourish Bowl with Coconut Tzatziki

Serves 4
Prep: 1 hour 20 minutes
Cook: 10–15 minutes

Marinade

1 tbsp miso paste

2 tbsp mirin

1 tsp soy sauce

1 tbsp fresh ginger, grated

1 red chilli, seeds removed,
  finely chopped

water/extra-virgin olive oil,
  to thin if needed

Tofu

200 g firm tofu, cut into strips/
  cubes

extra-virgin olive oil, for cooking

Salad

2 cups zucchini noodles or
  ribbons/shredded cabbage/
  baby spinach leaves

½ cup edamame

1 cup brown rice/quinoa,
  cooked

1 avocado, seed and skin
  removed, cubed

½ cup kimchi

2 sheets nori, roughly torn

sesame seeds, to serve

Coconut Tzatziki

150 g plain coconut yoghurt

1 small cucumber, grated,
  moisture squeezed out

1 tbsp lemon juice/apple
  cider vinegar

2–4 tbsp extra-virgin
  olive oil

2–4 tbsp fresh herbs (e.g.
  mint, chives etc), chopped

1–2 garlic cloves, crushed

sea salt and pepper,
  to taste

In a small bowl, whisk together the marinade ingredients.

Place the tofu in a bowl, then pour over the marinade ingredients. Cover and refrigerate for 30–60 minutes.

To make the coconut tzatziki, mix all of the ingredients in a bowl and season to taste, then set aside in the fridge.

Heat the extra-virgin olive oil in a frying pan over a medium-high heat, then add the tofu and cook on each side for 2 minutes or until lightly golden. Alternatively, heat the oven to 180°C and line a baking tray with baking paper. Place the tofu on the tray and cook for 10 minutes or until lightly golden.

To assemble, place the shredded red cabbage, zucchini noodles or ribbons, spinach leaves, edamame, brown rice, avocado and kimchi in a bowl. Top with the ginger tofu, nori and sesame seeds. Dress with the tzatziki dressing.

—

Kimchi is a great addition to support your gut health because, as a fermented food, it contains live probiotics. Miso paste is available from the Asian section of major supermarkets, Asian grocery stores or health food stores.

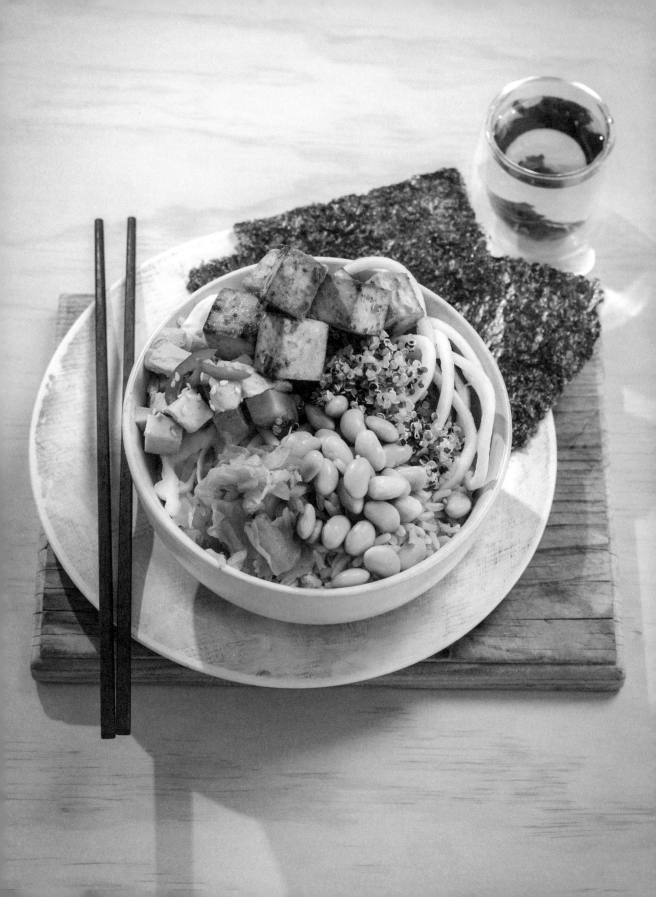

GF, V • **Antioxidants**

Chilled Beetroot Soup

Serves 2–3
Prep: 5 minutes
Cook: 45 minutes

Soup

4 medium beetroots

1 L water/miso stock
(1 tbsp gluten-free miso paste
to 1 cup water)

1–2 garlic cloves

1 tbsp beetroot powder, optional

500 g natural yoghurt

1 tbsp lemon juice

2 tbsp tahini

sea salt, to taste

Topping

drizzle tahini

½ bunch spring onion, finely
chopped

1–2 tbsp dill, chopped

1–2 tbsp walnuts, crushed

Place the beetroots in a medium pot and cover with water. Bring to the boil and simmer until tender. Place the beetroots and cooking water in the fridge until cool. Once cool, grate finely.

In a blender, add the beetroots, cooking water, garlic, beetroot powder, yoghurt, lemon juice, tahini and salt.

Pour into a bowl and top with a drizzle of tahini, spring onion, dill and walnuts.

—

To support gut health, powdered probiotics can be added to this soup before blending.

GF, V • Antioxidants

Golden Beetroot Carpaccio with Micro Herbs

Serves 4
Prep: 20 minutes
  (+ 60 minutes curing time)
Cook: n/a

3 tbsp extra-virgin olive oil

2 tbsp orange juice

1 tsp red wine vinegar

½ tsp cumin, ground

salt and pepper, to taste

2–4 medium red/golden
  beetroots, peeled

1 packet micro herbs

50 g goat's cheese, crumbled

2 tbsp toasted macadamia nuts,
  chopped

In a small bowl, whisk together the extra-virgin olive oil, orange juice, red wine vinegar, cumin, salt and pepper. Adjust seasoning to suit.

Very thinly and gently slice the beetroots using a mandolin or sharp knife. Add to a large bowl, pour in the dressing and mix well. Leave to cure for 30–60 minutes, or longer if desired.

Arrange the beetroot slices in a circular shape, with slices overlapping, on 1 large serving platter or individual plates. Drizzle over any remaining dressing and top with the micro herbs, goat's cheese and macadamia nuts.

—

Golden beetroot tends to have a slightly sweeter and less earthy flavour compared to red beetroot. Golden beetroots are still a good source of antioxidants.

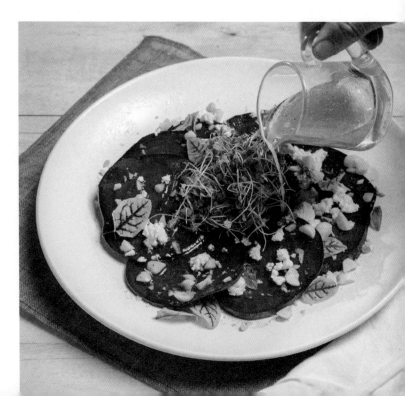

GF • **Healthy fats**

Lemon Chicken & Avocado Caesar Salad

Serves 2–4
Prep: 15 minutes
Cook: 10 minutes

Dressing

1 small avocado, seed and skin removed

1 tbsp extra-virgin olive oil

1 tbsp lemon juice

1 garlic clove, crushed

2–4 tbsp Greek yoghurt

sea salt and pepper, to taste

Salad

250 g chicken thigh, trimmed

2 tbsp lemon juice

1 tsp lemon zest

¼ cup lemon thyme, finely chopped

2 tbsp extra-virgin olive oil + 1 tbsp for cooking

½–1 tsp sea salt

1 tsp pepper, ground

2 cups baby cos lettuce

3 eggs, boiled and chopped

¼ cup parmesan cheese, shaved

To make the dressing, add all of the ingredients to a blender and blend until smooth, then adjust seasoning to suit.

In a bowl, mix together the chicken, lemon juice, zest, lemon thyme, extra-virgin olive oil, salt and pepper. Preheat the extra-virgin olive oil in a frying pan, add the chicken and cook on each side for approximately 3 minutes, or until cooked through. Remove from the pan and let sit for 5 minutes before slicing.

In a large mixing bowl, add the baby cos lettuce, eggs, parmesan and dressing.

Place the salad onto a plate, then top with the sliced chicken and a drizzle of extra dressing if desired.

—

This dressing also doubles as a creamy dip. Pair with veggies and seed crackers as a healthy snack.

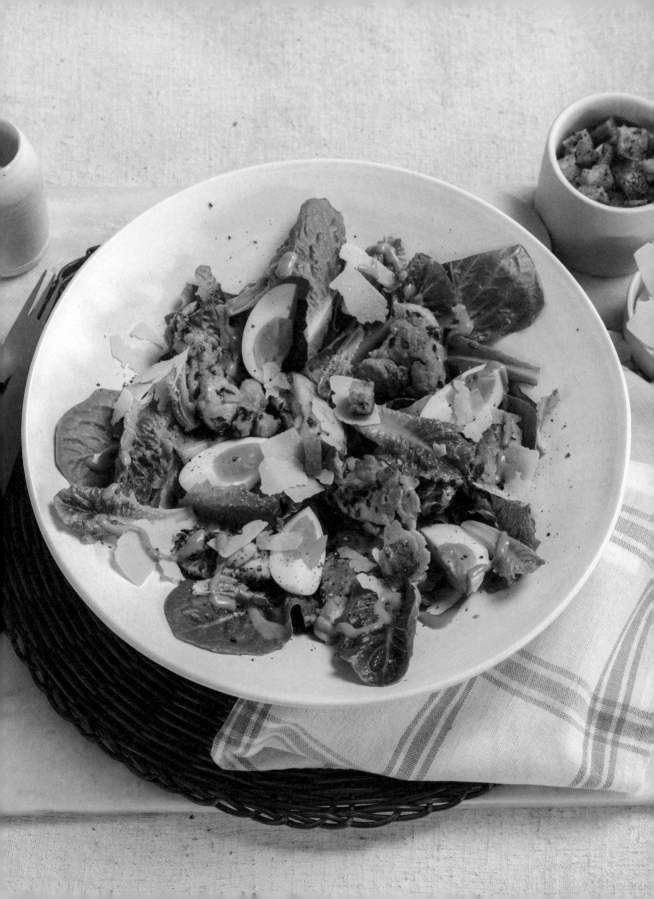

GF, V • **Vitamin C**

Middle Eastern Halloumi & Tofu Veggie Bake

Serves 2
Prep: 15 minutes
Cook: 25 minutes

Dressing

40 g Greek yoghurt

1 tbsp lemon juice

½ tsp cumin, ground

½ tsp raw honey

Veggie Bake

75 g firm tofu, cut into strips

1 bunch broccolini, cut into thin florets

½ red onion, peeled and sliced

15 mL extra-virgin olive oil, for cooking

¼ tsp coriander seeds, ground

¼ tsp cinnamon, ground

¼ tsp allspice, ground

75 g halloumi, cut into strips

150 g cherry/grape tomatoes

½ bunch parsley, finely chopped

2 tbsp macadamia nuts

Preheat the oven to 180°C and line a baking tray with baking paper.

To make the dressing, combine all of the ingredients in a small bowl. Mix well and set aside.

In a large bowl, combine the tofu, broccolini and red onion. Drizzle with the extra-virgin olive oil and the spices and mix well.

Spread the veggies and tofu in a single layer over the tray.

Bake for 10 minutes. Turn the veggies and tofu, add the halloumi and tomatoes to the pan and cook for a further 15 minutes or until the halloumi is cooked.

Remove from the oven, divide between 2 plates and sprinkle with the parsley and macadamia nuts. Drizzle with the yoghurt dressing.

—

As a dressing alternative, replace yoghurt with tahini and add a splash of water. Tahini is a source of plant-based calcium, iron, copper and manganese.

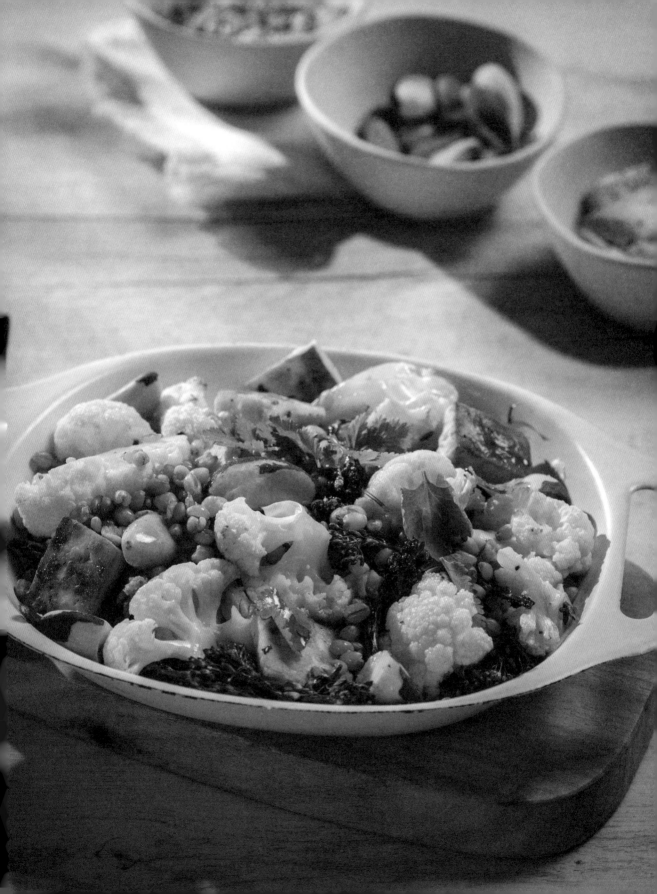

GF, V • **Beta-carotene**

Rainbow Legume Pasta Salad

Serves 2
Prep: 10 minutes
Cook: 20 minutes

Pasta Sauce

2 tbsp extra-virgin olive oil

1 small carrot, peeled and finely diced

¼ red capsicum, seeds removed, finely diced

½ cup grape/cherry tomatoes, halved

1 cup leftover roasted veggies (e.g. pumpkin, sweet potato etc)

Salad

1 cup legume pasta, cooked

¼ cup parmesan cheese/ cheese of your choice

1 tbsp hemp seeds

In a frying pan heat the extra-virgin olive oil. Add the carrot, capsicum and tomatoes, then cook until tender and the tomatoes have broken down. Stir in the leftover roasted veggies and slightly crush the mixture to the desired sauce consistency.

Remove from the heat and let cool.

Stir the sauce through the leftover cooked pasta, then add the parmesan and sprinkle with the hemp seeds.

Add optional extras like feta cheese, tuna, chicken, tofu or salmon.

—

For a dairy-free version, try sneaking some crumbled firm tofu into the sauce and sprinkling with nutritional yeast. This recipe is popular with fussy eaters.

V • Fibre

Crushed Pea Bruschetta with Avocado & Goat's Cheese Salsa

Serves 4
Prep: 15 minutes
Cook: 5 minutes

Bruschetta

4 slices sourdough bread

1 tbsp extra-virgin olive oil

Salsa

1 avocado, seed and skin removed, diced into 2 cm pieces

1 tbsp lemon juice

1–2 large Roma tomatoes/ ½ punnet cherry tomatoes, diced

50 g goat's cheese, lightly crumbled

sea salt and pepper, to taste

Crushed Peas

1 cup green peas, cooked and cooled

½ tsp spirulina powder, optional

¼ bunch fresh mint leaves

1–2 tbsp extra-virgin olive oil

salt and pepper, to taste

1 tbsp lemon juice

Drizzle the bread with the extra-virgin olive oil. Place under a grill until lightly toasted, then set aside.

To make the salsa, combine the avocado, lemon juice, tomato and goat's cheese in a bowl. Season to taste, then set aside.

To make the crushed peas, combine all of the ingredients in a food processor and pulse until the mixture comes together.

Spread the crushed pea mixture onto slices of toasted bread and top with the salsa. Serve immediately.

—

Spirulina is a source of vitamin K which is important for bone health, something menopausal women need to be mindful of due to a decrease in oestrogen levels. Spirulina can be purchased in the health section of major supermarkets, at health food stores or chemists.

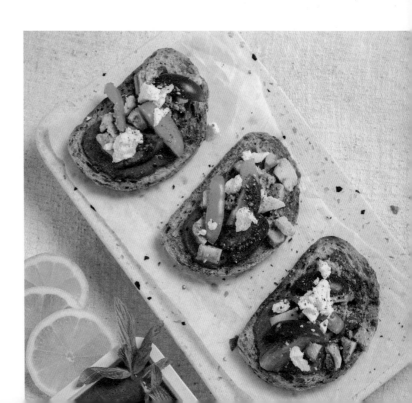

DF, GF, V • Vitamin C

Dairy-Free Pesto, Potato & Egg Salad

Serves 4–6
Prep: 15 minutes
Cook: 30 minutes

Pesto

1 bunch basil leaves

2 garlic cloves, crushed

½ cup nutritional yeast

¼ cup cashews, toasted

juice of 1 lemon

¼ cup extra-virgin olive oil

Salad

750 g new potatoes, halved

4 eggs

2 cups baby spinach leaves

1 bunch parsley, finely chopped

1 punnet cherry tomatoes

To make the pesto, blend all of the ingredients in a food processor until smooth, then set aside.

In a large saucepan or steamer, add the potatoes and water and boil or steam for 10 minutes or until tender. Drain and leave to cool.

In a small saucepan, add the eggs and water. Bring to the boil and cook for 3 minutes. Remove the eggs and leave to cool. Once cooled, peel and cut the eggs into quarters.

In a large bowl, mix together the potatoes, pesto, spinach, parsley and tomatoes. Spoon onto a serving dish and top with the eggs.

—

Nutritional yeast is a great vegan and non-dairy substitute for parmesan. It has a cheesy and nutty flavour, is a good source of protein and is rich in B vitamins.

GF, V • **Protein**

Savoury Baked Ricotta & Goat's Cheese with Roasted Veggies

Serves 5 as a snack or 2 as a meal
Prep: 10 minutes
Cook: 30 minutes

300 g fresh ricotta cheese

1 egg, beaten

100 g goat's cheese

1 cup roasted vegetables
  (e.g. capsicum, eggplant,
  sundried tomatoes,
  zucchini etc)

¼ cup olives, sliced

¼ cup fresh herbs of your
  choice, finely chopped

pinch chilli flakes, optional

2 tbsp pine nuts

2 tsp extra-virgin olive oil

Preheat the oven to 180°C and line a small square baking tray with baking paper.

In a mixing bowl, combine the ricotta, egg, goat's cheese, veggies, olives, herbs, chilli and pine nuts.

Spoon the mixture into a medium baking dish or individual ramekins, then drizzle with the extra-virgin olive oil.

Bake for 15–30 minutes, depending on baking dish size, or until lightly golden on top.

Let sit until slightly cooled, then remove from the baking dish or ramekins and cut into slices or wedges.

—

As a simple balanced lunch, serve this ricotta on top of good-quality sourdough or seeded bread topped with rocket leaves.

DF, GF • Selenium

Prawn, Watermelon & Cashew Lettuce Cups with Coconut Avocado Dressing

Serves 6–8
Prep: 20 minutes
Cook: n/a

Coconut Avocado Dressing

1 avocado, seed and skin
   removed, diced

½ cup coconut milk + extra
   if needed

1 red chilli, seeds removed,
   sliced

1 tbsp lime juice

1 garlic clove, crushed

1 tbsp tamari soy sauce,
   gluten-free

1–2 tsp fish sauce, gluten-free

water/extra-virgin olive oil, to
   thin if needed

Lettuce Cups

1–2 cups watermelon, rind
   removed, finely diced

½ cup cashews, roughly crushed

1–2 red chillies, seeds removed,
   sliced + extra to serve

½ bunch coriander leaves,
   chopped + extra to serve

1–2 baby cos lettuce, leaves
   separated

500 g cooked prawns, peeled
   and deveined

To make the dressing, combine all of the ingredients in a food processor or blender, adding extra coconut milk until desired consistency is reached. Adjust seasoning to suit. Set aside in the fridge.

Combine the watermelon, cashews, chilli and coriander in a small bowl. Top each lettuce leaf with 1–2 prawns, the watermelon mixture and coconut avocado dressing. Finish with the extra chilli slices and fresh coriander.

—

Prawns are a good source of minerals zinc and iodine, both important for thyroid health.

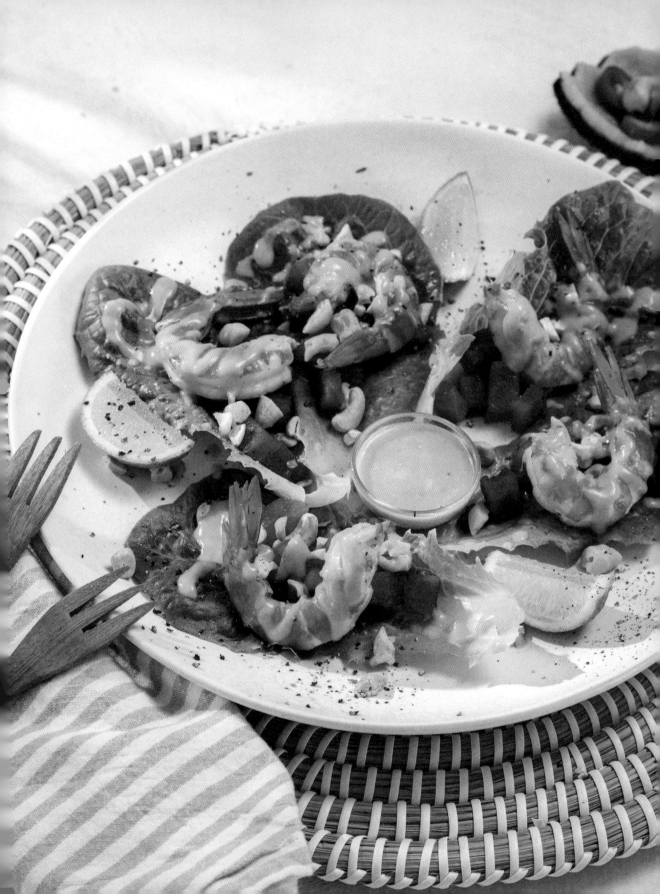

GF, V • **Protein**

Quinoa, Herb, Pea & Ricotta Frittata

Serves 10–12
Prep: 10 minutes
Cook: 25 minutes

8 eggs

2 garlic cloves, crushed

150 g fresh ricotta cheese

100 g feta/goat's cheese, crumbled

¾ cup quinoa, cooked and cooled

1 cup green peas, frozen and thawed

¼ cup basil, finely chopped

½ bunch spring onions, finely chopped

salt and pepper, to taste

Preheat the oven to 180°C.

Place 10–12 patty pans into a muffin tin.

In a large mixing bowl, whisk the eggs and garlic and then add the ricotta, feta or goat's cheese, quinoa, peas, basil, spring onions, salt and pepper.

Spoon the mixture into individual patty pans and cook in the oven for 20–25 minutes or until just set and slightly golden on top.

—

For a dairy-free version still rich in calcium, swap the cheese for crumbled firm tofu (calcium-set) and a sprinkle of nutritional yeast. Get kids involved in this recipe by asking them to whisk the ingredients together.

GF, V • **Vitamin C**

Roasted Capsicum & Almond Soup

Serves 4
Prep: 30 minutes
Cook: 30 minutes

Soup

2 yellow capsicums

2 red capsicums

1 tbsp extra-virgin olive oil

1 small brown onion, peeled
   and finely sliced

2 cloves of garlic

4 sprigs fresh thyme

2 sprigs fresh rosemary

1 cup almonds, skin on and
   roasted, roughly chopped

500 mL miso stock (1 tbsp of
   gluten-free miso paste to
   250 mL hot water)

Serve With

chopped parsley

2 tbsp feta cheese, crumbled

Preheat the grill. Place the capsicums on a baking tray, then grill for 5 minutes each side or until the skin is blackened. Once blackened, place the capsicum in a bowl and cover to sweat and cool. Once cooled, remove the skin and seeds and roughly chop.

In a large saucepan, add the extra-virgin olive oil and onion, sauté for 10 minutes or until golden brown. Add the garlic and herbs, then further cook for 5 minutes. Stir in the capsicum, almonds and stock, and bring to a simmer for 10 minutes.

Blend until smooth and serve topped with the parsley and feta.

—

Using almonds with the skin on is a great way to add more prebiotic fibre into your diet. Prebiotic fibre is fuel for gut bacteria, helping to support a healthy gut. Miso paste is available from the Asian section of major supermarkets, Asian grocery stores or health food stores.

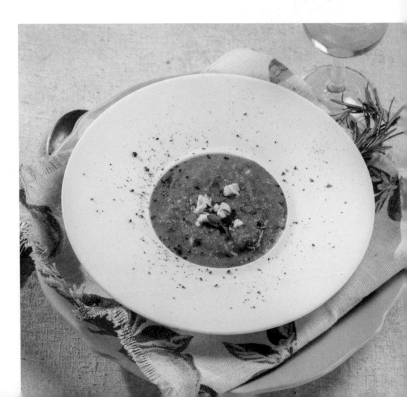

DF • **Vitamin B6**

Super Sausage & Mushroom Rolls

Serves 2–4
Prep: 20 minutes
Cook: 20–30 minutes

2 tbsp maca powder

2 tsp fennel seeds

1 tsp cumin seeds

¼ tsp nutmeg, ground

1 tsp ginger, ground

2 tbsp wholemeal breadcrumbs

150 g pork mince

1 tsp fresh ginger, grated

2 garlic cloves, crushed

1 bunch sage, chopped

2 tbsp honey

150 g mushrooms, finely chopped

100 g zucchini, finely grated, excess water squeezed out

2 eggs, whisked + 1 extra for brushing

2 tsp sea salt and pepper, to taste

2 sheets of puff pastry

2 tbsp chia seeds

Preheat the oven to 200°C.

To a large mixing bowl add the maca powder, fennel seeds, cumin seeds, nutmeg, ginger, wholemeal breadcrumbs, pork mince, ginger, garlic, sage, honey, mushrooms and zucchini, and mix well. Add 2 eggs and season with salt and pepper, then combine well.

Lay the puff pastry sheets out and divide the meat mixture between the 2 sheets, placing the mixture in the middle of each sheet. Fold the pastry over and seal along the edges.

Brush the top with the remaining egg, whisked, to give it a shine. Sprinkle the top with chia seeds.

Bake the sausage rolls for 20 minutes or until the centre of the rolls reaches 60°C.

Take out of the oven. Cut the sausage rolls into quarters to serve.

—

This recipe is a great way to sneak in a few extra veggies! For a vegetarian version, crumbled tofu can be used in place of the pork mince. Maca powder can be purchased in the health section of major supermarkets, at health food stores or chemists.

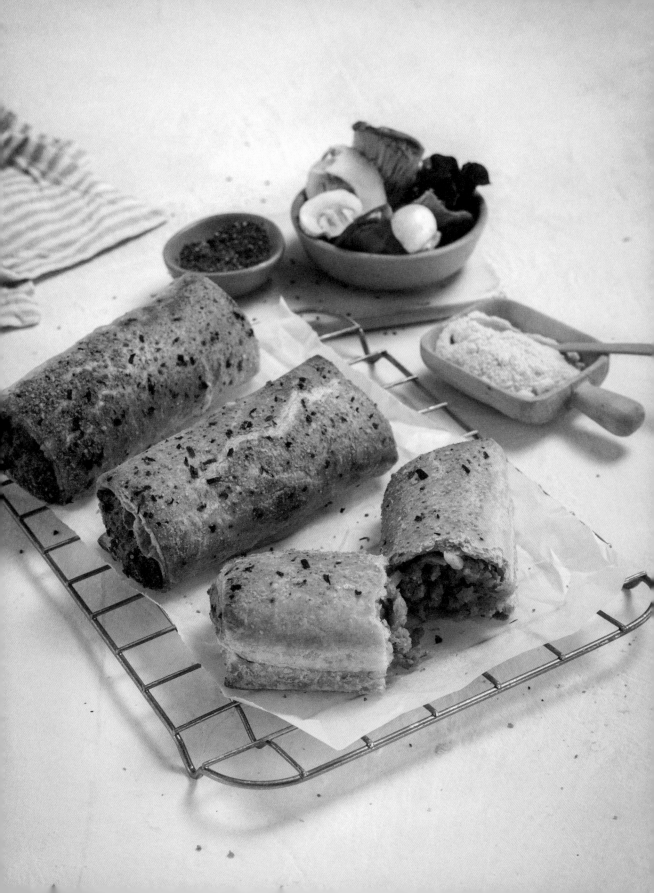

DF, GF • Zinc

Thai Salmon Salad

Serves 2
Prep: 15 minutes
Cook: 10 minutes

Protein

150 g salmon fillet

5 mL extra-virgin olive oil

1 tsp sea salt

1 tsp pepper, ground

Dressing

2–4 tbsp extra-virgin olive oil

1 long red chilli, seeds removed, thinly sliced + extra to serve

¼ cup mint leaves, torn + extra to serve

1–2 tbsp fish sauce, gluten-free

juice of 1 lime

½ tsp raw honey

Salad

2 cups mixed salad leaves

1 small avocado, seed and skin removed, diced

1 small red onion, thinly sliced

100 g grape tomatoes, halved

¼ cup roasted macadamia nuts/cashews, chopped

Season the salmon with the extra-virgin olive oil, salt and pepper. Sear on each side for a few minutes, until cooked to your liking, then remove from the heat. Cut the salmon into thin slices and add to a large bowl.

In a small bowl, whisk together the extra-virgin olive oil, chilli, mint leaves, fish sauce, lime juice and honey. Pour this dressing over the salmon and add the mixed salad leaves, avocado, onion and tomatoes. Gently toss.

Place the salad onto a plate and scatter with the extra chilli, mint leaves and toasted macadamia nuts.

—

If you are very active, add a serve of rice or cooked soba noodles to this dish to support recovery and energy levels.

GF, V • **Protein**

Turmeric, Sicilian Olive & Parmesan Loaf

Serves 6–8
Prep: 15 minutes
Cook: 30 minutes

200 g almond meal

50 g coconut flour

1½ tsp baking powder

1 tsp turmeric, ground

1 tsp sea salt

¼ tsp pepper

4 large/5 medium eggs

2 tbsp extra-virgin olive oil

¼ cup water

2–4 tbsp Sicilian green olives,
pitted and sliced

100 g parmesan cheese,
grated/nutritional yeast

1 tsp dried rosemary

Preheat the oven to 180°C and line a loaf tin with baking paper.

In a large bowl, combine the almond meal, coconut flour, baking powder, turmeric, salt and pepper. Mix well.

In a small bowl, whisk together the eggs, extra-virgin olive oil and water.

Add the wet mix to the dry mix and combine well. Stir in the olives and parmesan.

Pour the mixture into the prepared loaf in and sprinkle with the dried rosemary.

Place in the oven for 20–30 minutes until lightly golden on top, and when a skewer is inserted, it comes out clean.

—

As a nourishing lunch, serve a slice of this loaf topped with avocado and a veggie-rich side salad.

DF, GF, V, VG • **Vitamin C**

Asian Roasted Pumpkin Soup with Quinoa & Toasted Coconut

Serves 4–6
Prep: 10 minutes
Cook: 40 minutes

1–2 tbsp extra-virgin olive oil

1 leek, finely sliced

2 garlic cloves, peeled and
  halved

1 tsp turmeric, ground/fresh

1 red chilli, seeds removed,
  finely sliced

1 tsp ginger, ground/fresh

750 g pumpkin, diced and
  pre-roasted

½ cup quinoa, uncooked

400 mL can coconut milk

1 bunch coriander, chopped
  + reserve a small amount
  to serve

1 L vegetable stock, gluten-free

⅓ cup coconut chips

salt and pepper, to taste

Heat the extra-virgin olive oil in a large saucepan over medium heat. Add the leek and cook for 5 minutes until softened, trying not to brown. Add the garlic, turmeric, ginger, half of the chilli and fry off for 1–2 minutes before adding the pumpkin and quinoa. Mix well.

Add the coconut milk, coriander and enough stock to cover, then bring to a gentle simmer and cook for 30 minutes, or until the quinoa is cooked.

Blend the mixture with a stick blender until the desired consistency is reached, then season with salt and pepper.

Ladle into bowls and top with the extra coriander, remaining chilli and toasted coconut chips.

—

Quinoa has a higher protein content compared to other grains. It is a great choice for vegetarians looking to increase their protein intake.

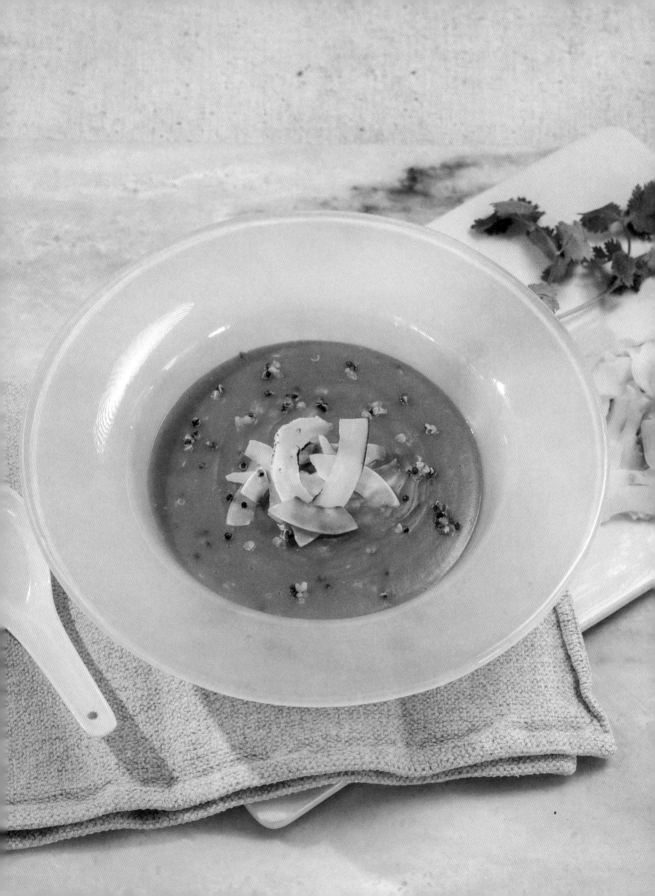

Dinner

DF, GF • **Healthy fats**

Cashew-Crumbed Salmon Lettuce Cups

Serves 4
Prep: 15 minutes
Cook: 10 minutes

Salmon

¼ cup cashews, crushed

¾ cup wholemeal breadcrumbs (gluten-free if required)

1 tbsp lime zest

400 g salmon fillet, skin removed, cut into 2–3 cm cubes

1 egg, lightly beaten

1 tbsp virgin coconut oil/ extra-virgin olive oil

For Serving

1 cos lettuce, separated into small cups

1 small bag kale slaw, premade

1 tub tzatziki/hummus, optional

In a food processor combine the cashews, breadcrumbs and lime zest. Pour into a bowl.

Dip each salmon piece in the beaten egg, then transfer to the breadcrumb bowl and cover with the breadcrumb mixture, patting gently to help the crumbs stick.

Heat the oil in a frying or griddle pan over a medium heat. Cook the salmon pieces on each side until lightly golden or cooked to your liking.

Top the lettuce cups with the kale slaw, a dollop of tzatziki or hummus and the salmon.

—

For a nut-free option, swap cashews for sesame seeds for the same phytoestrogen benefits.

DF, GF • **Antioxidants**

Extra-Virgin Olive Oil Poached Fish with Roasted Nut, Citrus & Micro Herb Salad

Serves 4
Prep: 15 minutes
Cook: 20–30 minutes

Poached Fish

4 × 150 g firm fish fillets/
  1 large fillet, skin off, at room
  temperature

2 garlic cloves, finely chopped

1 tsp whole black peppercorns

a few sprigs fresh rosemary/
  herbs of your choice

200–400 mL extra-virgin
  olive oil/miso stock (1 tbsp
  gluten-free miso paste to
  250 mL water)

Salad

1 pink grapefruit, peeled and
  segmented

1 orange, peeled and
  segmented

1 container micro herbs

1–2 small radish, thinly sliced

⅓ cup roasted nuts of choice,
  chopped

1–2 tbsp extra-virgin olive oil

salt and pepper, to taste

Place the salmon, garlic, pepper and rosemary into a deep saucepan in a single layer. Pour over the extra-virgin olive oil until it just covers the salmon.

Poach over a low heat (70–80°C) for 20–30 minutes or until the salmon easily flakes apart. Remove the salmon from the oil and drain on paper towel.

To make the salad, gently combine all of the ingredients in a small bowl, then drizzle with the extra-virgin olive oil, salt and pepper.

Serve the salad on top of or alongside the salmon.

—

Rosemary aids healthy oestrogen metabolism and may assist with estrogenic type symptoms.

DF, GF • Protein

Baked Barramundi with Honey Carrots

Serves 4
Prep: 15 minutes
Cook: 15 minutes

400 g Dutch/regular carrots, halved lengthways

1 tbsp raw honey, melted

1–2 tsp lemon zest

2–4 tbsp extra-virgin olive oil + extra to drizzle

4 × 150 g barramundi fillets, skin removed

sea salt and pepper

sesame seeds, toasted

Preheat the oven to 180°C. Line a baking tray with baking paper.

In a large bowl, combine the carrots, honey, lemon zest and extra-virgin olive oil. Toss well.

Spread the carrots onto the baking tray and top with the barramundi fillets, then drizzle with the extra-virgin olive oil and season.

Place in the oven for 15 minutes or until the barramundi is cooked to your liking and the carrots are tender.

Remove from the oven and sprinkle with the sesame seeds.

—

Serve with a leafy green salad for added antioxidant support.

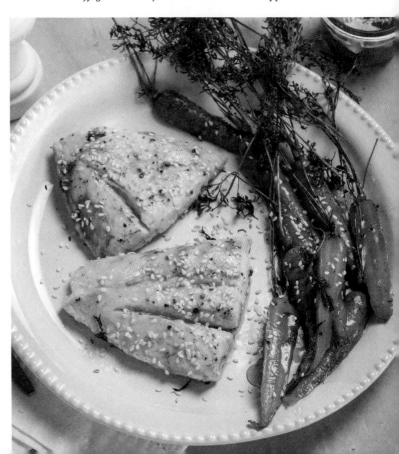

DF, GF, V, VG • **Vitamin C**

Chargrilled Vegetable Skewers with Cashew Dipping Sauce

Serves 2–3
Prep: 20 minutes
Cook: 10 minutes

Spicy Cashew Dipping Sauce

¼ cup raw cashews

1 tbsp extra-virgin olive oil

1 tbsp fish sauce, gluten-free
  (omit for vegetarian/vegan)

1 tbsp tamari soy sauce,
  gluten-free

1 tbsp honey/maple syrup

juice of 1 lime

2 tbsp water

Skewers

10 skewers

2 zucchini, cut into 1–2 cm
  rounds

1 punnet grape tomatoes

1 yellow capsicum, seeds
  removed, cut into evenly sized
  square pieces

1 bunch asparagus, cut into
  equal-length batons

extra-virgin olive oil, for cooking

Serving Suggestion

rocket, pine nut and parmesan
  salad

Soak wooden skewers prior to cooking.

To make the sauce, combine the cashews, extra-virgin olive oil, fish sauce, soy sauce, honey and lime juice in a blender with enough water to make a runny consistency. Set aside until needed.

Thread the vegetables onto the pointy end of a skewer. Preheat a barbecue or grill plate with the extra-virgin olive oil and place the skewers on the grill. Cook for 7 minutes or until the vegetables are charred and tender. Take off the heat and serve with the cashew sauce.

—

This recipe is a delicious starter or light meal rich in healthy fats. In fact, the healthy fat content of the spicy cashew dipping sauce will help increase the absorption of vitamins and antioxidants from the vegetables.

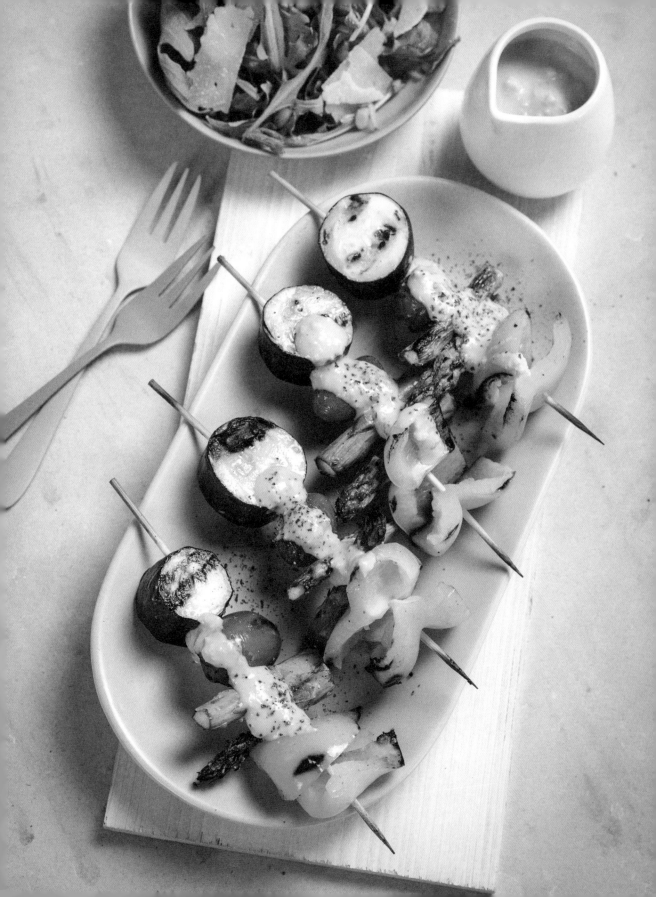

DF, GF • **Vitamin B6**

Chicken Biryani with Coconut Yoghurt Dressing

Serves 2
Prep: 15 minutes
Cook: 30 minutes

To Serve

coriander leaves

2 tbsp flaked almonds

Coconut Yoghurt Dressing

70 g coconut yoghurt

2 tbsp extra-virgin olive oil

2 tbsp coriander, finely chopped

1 tbsp lemon juice

½–1 tsp sea salt/tamari soy
sauce, gluten-free

Chicken Biryani

20 mL extra-virgin olive oil

150 g chicken thigh, trimmed
and cut into chunks

1 small brown onion, peeled
and diced

1 garlic clove, crushed

1 tbsp fresh ginger, grated

1 tsp garam masala

1 tsp turmeric, ground

1 tsp cumin, ground

½ tsp cinnamon, ground

½ tsp sea salt

½ tsp black pepper

200 g cauliflower rice

125 mL water/chicken stock,
gluten-free + extra if needed

To make the dressing, combine all of the ingredients in a small bowl, then mix well and set aside in the fridge.

Heat the extra-virgin olive oil to a medium-high heat in a frying pan. Add the chicken and brown. Remove from the pan.

Add the onion to the pan and cook for 3 minutes, before adding the garlic and ginger. After a minute, add the remaining spices and fry off for 1 minute. Return the chicken to the pan and cook for 10 minutes or until cooked through.

Add the cauliflower rice to the pan and combine well. Add enough stock to cover, then place the lid back on the pan and simmer for 5 minutes or until the cauliflower rice has softened. Season to taste.

Remove from the pan and spoon into serving bowls. Top with the coconut yoghurt dressing, coriander leaves and a sprinkle of flaked almonds.

—

Cauliflower rice can be alternated with broccoli rice. Both belong to the brassica family and contain sulforaphane, a type of phytochemical which has potent antioxidant effects and may help to promote detoxification and liver health.

DF, GF • **Healthy fats**

Warm Salmon & Zucchini Noodle Salad with Spicy Cashew Dressing

Serves 2
Prep: 15 minutes
Cook: 8 minutes

Spicy Cashew Dressing

25 g raw cashews

10 mL extra-virgin olive oil

1 tbsp fish sauce, gluten-free

1 tbsp tamari soy sauce, gluten-free

1–2 tsp raw honey

juice of 1 lime

water, to thin

Noodle Salad

5 mL extra-virgin olive oil

2 × 100 g salmon fillets

2 small zucchini, cut into spirals, blanched and patted dry

150 g grape/cherry tomatoes, halved

50 g avocado, seed and skin removed, diced

½ bunch coriander, stems removed, chopped + extra to serve

3 red chillies, seeds removed, julienned + extra to serve

To make the spicy dressing, in a blender, thoroughly combine the cashews, extra-virgin olive oil, fish sauce, soy sauce, honey, lime juice and enough water to make a runny consistency. Adjust the seasoning to suit, then set aside.

Preheat a frying pan with a drizzle of extra-virgin olive oil, then add the salmon and cook on each side for a few minutes or until cooked to your liking.

In a large bowl, add the zucchini, tomatoes, avocado, coriander and half of the dressing, mix well.

Top with the salmon and finish with a drizzle of dressing, freshly sliced chilli and coriander.

—

Use half rice noodles and half zucchini noodles if preferred.

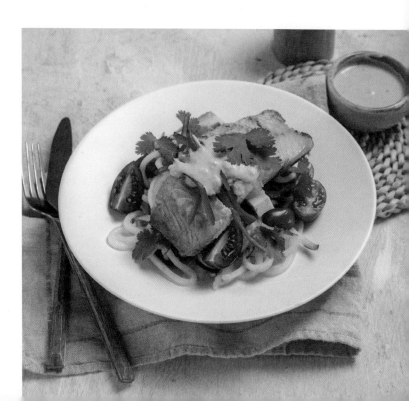

DF, GF • **Protein**

Warm Ginger Satay Chicken Salad with Turmeric Cauliflower

Serves 2
Prep: 15 minutes
Cook: 50 minutes

Turmeric Cauliflower

1–2 tsp virgin coconut oil

1–2 garlic cloves, crushed

¼ tsp turmeric, ground/grated

sea salt and pepper, to taste

2 cups cauliflower, cut into florets

½ tbsp lime juice

Peanut Satay Sauce

1 tbsp natural peanut butter

1 tbsp lime juice

2 tbsp water

½ tbsp raw honey

1 tsp miso paste, gluten-free

½ tsp chilli, seeds removed, chopped/flakes

Ginger Chicken

1–2 tbsp virgin coconut oil, for cooking

250 g chicken breast, cut into strips

1 tbsp ginger, finely diced

1 garlic clove, crushed

1 tbsp tamari soy sauce, gluten-free

Assembly

½ cup cooked turmeric cauliflower

2 handfuls pea sprouts/ bean sprouts

½ cucumber, sliced

¼ bunch coriander, finely chopped

1 green chilli, seeds removed, sliced

¼ cup sesame seeds/ pumpkin seeds

For the turmeric cauliflower, heat the coconut oil in a small pan over a medium heat, then add in the garlic and cook for 1 minute. Add the turmeric, salt and pepper and stir until the cauliflower is fully coated with turmeric. Cover the pan with a lid and let cook for 2 minutes. Add the lime juice and stir to coat. Remove from heat and set aside.

For the peanut satay sauce, add all of the ingredients in a bowl and whisk until creamy and well combined.

To make the ginger chicken, add the chicken to a bowl with the ginger, garlic and tamari soy sauce, and mix well. Heat the coconut oil in a small pan over a medium heat, add the chicken and cook for 5 minutes on each side, or until cooked through.

To assemble, in each bowl, place the turmeric cauliflower in the bottom of a bowl, top with the chicken, pea or bean sprouts, cucumber, coriander, green chilli, seeds and drizzle with the peanut satay sauce.

—

Macadamia nut or almond butter can be used in place of peanut butter if preferred.

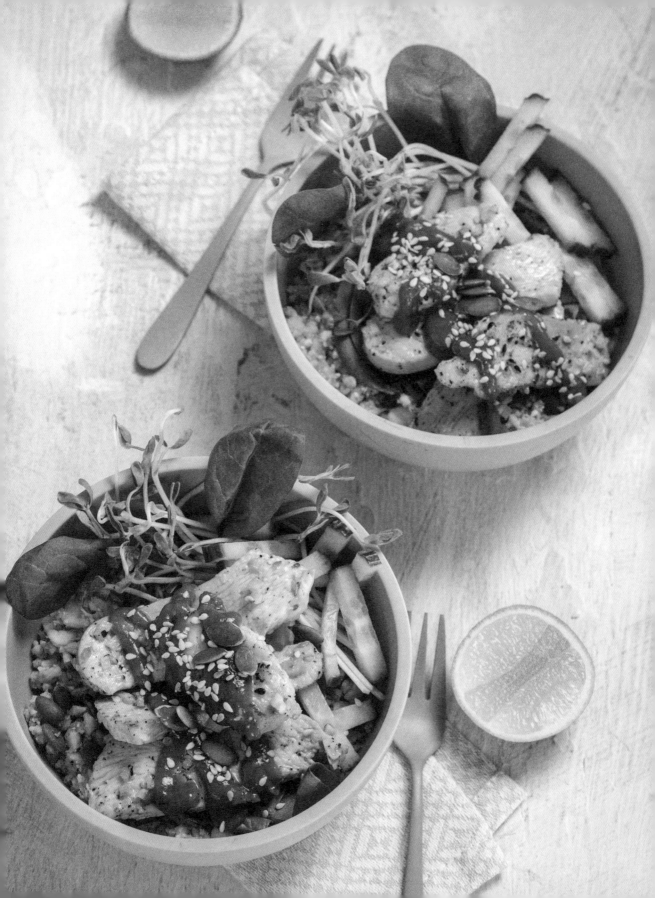

DF • **Protein**

Coconut Chicken Nuggets

Serves 4
Prep: 15 minutes
Cook: 10–15 minutes

1 cup wholemeal breadcrumbs

½ cup shredded coconut

2 tbsp fresh ginger, grated

1 tsp turmeric, ground

pinch black pepper and salt

2 eggs, lightly beaten

4 × 150 g chicken breasts,
  halved and lightly flattened

1 tbsp virgin coconut oil/
  extra-virgin olive oil + extra
  to serve

herbs of your choice, to serve

2 cups mixed lettuce leaves,
  to serve

lemon, quartered, to serve

In a bowl, mix the breadcrumbs, shredded coconut, ginger, turmeric, salt and pepper. In another bowl, mix the eggs.

Dip each chicken breast in the beaten egg and coat all over. Transfer to the breadcrumb bowl and cover with the breadcrumb mixture, patting gently to help the crumbs stick.

In a large frying pan add the oil and cook the chicken for approximately 5 minutes on each side, or until cooked through. Serve with the fresh herbs and mixed lettuce leaves, drizzled with the extra-virgin olive oil and a wedge of lemon.

—

If low on zinc, replace coconut with roughly ground pumpkin seeds. To get kids involved in this recipe, ask them to coat the chicken in the crumb mix.

GF, V • **Zinc**

Meatballs with Zucchini & Parmesan Salad

Serves 2
Prep: 15 minutes
Cook: 15 minutes

Meatballs

170–200 g beef mince/
  hard tofu, crumbled

1 egg, lightly beaten

1 shallot, peeled and finely cut

1 small beetroot, peeled and
  grated

½ bunch basil, finely chopped

1 garlic clove, crushed

½–1 tsp sea salt and pepper

5 mL extra-virgin olive oil

Salad

1 small avocado, seed and skin
  removed, sliced

1 medium zucchini, thinly sliced
  into rounds and blanched/
  lightly steamed

20 g goat's cheese, crumbled

30 g parmesan cheese, shaved

1 tbsp lemon juice

10 mL extra-virgin olive oil

10 g pine nuts, toasted

sea salt and pepper, to taste

In a bowl, combine the mince, egg, shallot, beetroot, basil, garlic, salt and pepper. Mix well and form into 2 cm balls.

Heat the olive oil in a frying pan over a medium heat. Add the meatballs and cook, turning every few minutes, until cooked through. Remove from the heat.

To make the salad, combine all of the ingredients in a bowl and mix well, then set aside.

Serve the meatballs on top of the salad.

—

Beetroot not only gives this dish colour, but is a delicious way to add extra antioxidants, potassium and folate.

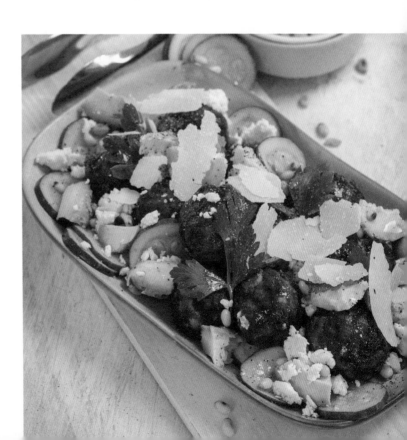

DF • **Vitamin B6**

Easy Ramen Noodle Soup with Miso Roasted Pork

Serves 1
Prep: 15 minutes
*   (+ 30 minutes marinating)*
Cook: 30 minutes

Miso Roasted Pork

100 g pork fillet

2 tsp soy sauce

2 tsp mirin

1 tsp light miso paste

1 tbsp sesame oil

Soup

1 packet ramen noodles
   (approximately 150 g)

¼ tbsp tamari soy sauce

¼ tbsp mirin

2 tsp fresh ginger, grated/sliced

250 mL bone broth stock
   (dissolve 2 tsp bone broth
   powder in 250 mL hot water)

Toppings

1 egg, soft boiled and halved

spring onion, chopped finely

nori/seaweed sheets

green/red chilli, seeds removed,
   thinly sliced

Combine the pork, soy sauce, mirin and miso. If time permits, marinate for 30 minutes.

Heat the sesame oil in a frying pan over a medium heat. Add the pork fillet, cook on each side for 4 minutes or until cooked through. Remove from the pan and let the pork rest before slicing thinly.

Bring a pot of water to the boil. Add the noodles and cook according to packet directions, then drain.

For the soup, place the soy sauce, mirin and ginger in a bowl. Add the prepared bone broth to the bowl and mix well, adjusting seasoning to suit.

Add the noodles, pork and egg to the bowl, followed by the spring onion, nori and chilli – or other toppings of your choice. Serve immediately.

—

For a vegetarian version, try tofu and shiitake mushrooms in place of pork and use miso in place of bone broth. Turmeric can be added to this broth for added anti-inflammatory support. Bone broth powder can be purchased in the health section of major supermarkets, at health food stores or chemists.

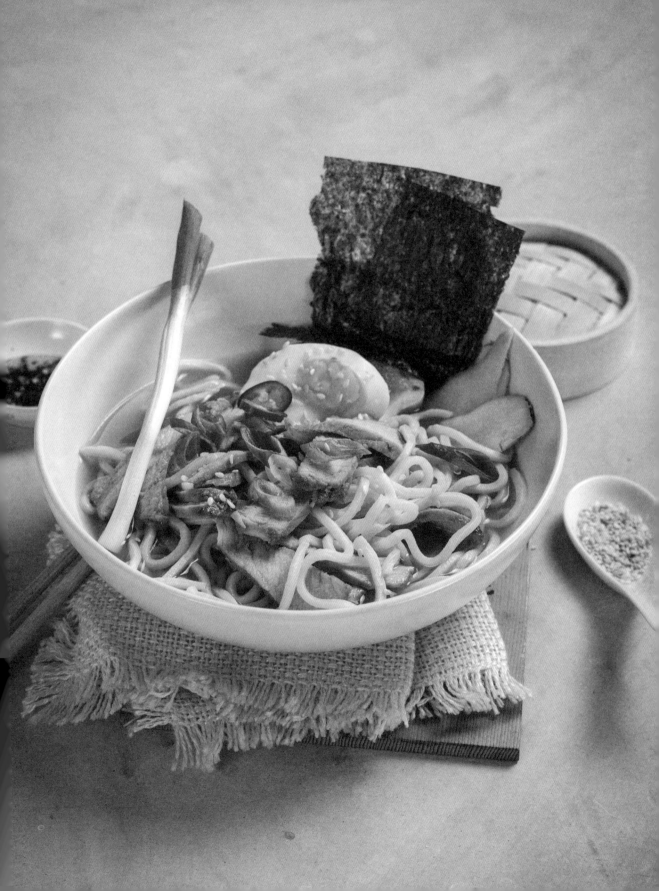

DF, GF, V, VG • **Vitamin C**

Green Curry with Tofu, Peas & Capsicum

Serves 4–6
Prep: 5 minutes
Cook: 20–30 minutes

1 tbsp extra-virgin olive oil

1 brown onion, finely sliced

1 tbsp ginger, grated

1 garlic clove, crushed

2 tbsp good-quality organic
   green curry paste

250–300 g firm tofu, cut into
   even-sized strips/cubes

1 red capsicum, seeds removed,
   finely sliced

400 mL coconut milk

250 mL vegetable stock,
   gluten-free

1 cup fresh/frozen green peas

100 g baby rocket leaves

steamed brown rice, to serve

1 bunch coriander, roughly
   chopped

In a frying pan or wok heat the extra-virgin olive oil, then add the onion and cook for 1 minute. Add the ginger and garlic, and cook until fragrant. Add the curry paste and stir-fry for 1 minute. Add the tofu and capsicum and cook for 2 minutes, then turn down the heat and pour in the coconut milk and enough stock to cover.

Gently simmer for 5 minutes. Stir in the peas and rocket, then take off the heat.

Serve with the steamed brown rice and coriander leaves.

—

Menopausal women should opt for calcium-set tofu as an easy way to boost calcium intake, while also getting the phytoestrogen benefits of soy products.

DF, GF • Vitamin C

Lamb & Macadamia Red Curry with Cauliflower Rice

Serves 2
Prep: 15 minutes
Cook: 1 hour 20 minutes

Curry

extra-virgin olive oil, for cooking

140 g diced lamb, trimmed

1 garlic clove, crushed

1 tbsp red curry paste

100 g red capsicum, seeds removed, sliced

2 small tomatoes, chopped

80 mL coconut milk

100 mL chicken stock, gluten-free + extra if needed

75 g baby spinach leaves

2 tbsp macadamia nuts, chopped + extra to serve

Cauliflower Rice

2 tsp extra-virgin olive oil

1 tsp turmeric, ground

¼ tsp pepper, ground

200 g cauliflower, blended into rice size/pre-bought

Heat the extra-virgin olive oil in a saucepan over a medium heat, add the lamb and brown for 2 minutes. Remove from the heat. Add the garlic and cook for 2 minutes, then add the curry paste to the pan and cook for a few minutes until fragrant.

Add the capsicum and tomatoes, fry off for 2 minutes before adding the lamb back to the pan.

Add the coconut milk and enough stock to cover the mixture. Cover with a lid and bring to a gentle simmer for approximately 60 minutes, until the meat is tender.

Once cooked stir through the spinach and macadamia nuts, before taking off the heat.

To make the cauliflower rice, heat the extra-virgin olive oil in a frying pan, add the turmeric and pepper and fry off for 1 minute. Add the cauliflower rice and stir-fry for a few minutes until golden in colour and tender.

Take off the heat and spoon into a bowl.

Top with the curry and finish with a sprinkle of macadamia nuts.

—

To increase your intake of fermented foods, replace chicken stock with miso stock, using 1 tsp Miso paste to 100 mL water. Miso paste is available from the Asian section of major supermarkets, Asian grocery stores or health food stores.

B vitamins

Mini Spicy Chicken, Beetroot & Goat's Cheese Pizza

Serves 4–8
Prep: 10 minutes
Cook: 20 minutes

1 container beetroot hummus

4–8 mini pizza bases/1 large pizza base, wholemeal/spelt

200–400 g chicken breast, cut into ½–1 cm strips

2 tbsp extra-virgin olive oil

salt and pepper, to taste

100 g button mushrooms, thinly sliced

1 small red onion, thinly sliced

1 green/red chilli, seeds removed, finely sliced

1 cup baby spinach/rocket leaves, finely chopped and drizzled with olive oil

100 g goat's cheese, crumbled

Preheat the oven to 180°C.

Spread the beetroot hummus over the pizza bases.

Place the chicken breast in a bowl and rub with the extra-virgin olive oil, sea salt and pepper until coated.

Place the chicken, mushroom, red onion and chilli evenly over the base. Drizzle with more oil, salt and pepper.

Place in the oven for approximately 15–20 minutes until the base is crispy and the chicken is cooked. Pull out of the oven, sprinkle with the baby spinach or rocket leaves and goat's cheese, and return to the oven for an additional 5 minutes.

—

Get kids involved in the process by asking them to 'decorate' their own pizzas. Regular hummus can be used as a base if preferred.

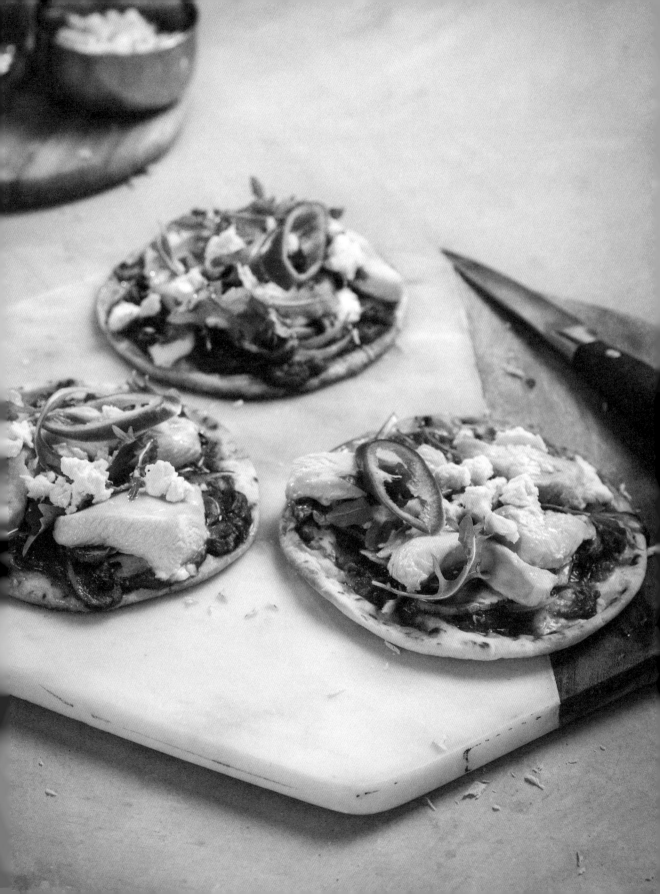

DF, GF • Zinc

Eye Fillet with Nut Salsa Verde & Charred Green Beans

Serves 2
Prep: 5 minutes
Cook: 20 minutes

Nut Salsa Verde

20 g pumpkin seeds, crushed

20 g pistachios, crushed

½ cup fresh coriander, stems removed, finely chopped

1 tbsp lemon zest

1 garlic clove, crushed

1 green chilli, seeds removed, thinly sliced

10 mL extra-virgin olive oil

salt and pepper, to taste

Eye Fillet and Beans

1 tbsp extra-virgin olive oil, for cooking

200 g eye fillet/sirloin steak/ hard tofu

1 cup green beans, trimmed

sea salt and pepper, to taste

To make the nut salsa verde, combine all of the ingredients in a bowl and mix well, set aside in the fridge.

In a frying pan or on a barbecue, heat a small splash of the extra-virgin olive oil over a medium-high heat and cook the steak to your liking. Remove from the heat, let rest and then cut into strips. Season to taste.

Meanwhile, drizzle a griddle pan or barbecue with a small splash of the extra-virgin olive oil, add the green beans and cook on each side until tender and slightly charred. Season to taste. Divide between 2 plates.

Arrange the steak next to the green beans and drizzle with the nut salsa verde.

—

Leftover nut salsa verde can be served with avocado on toast for a simple breakfast.

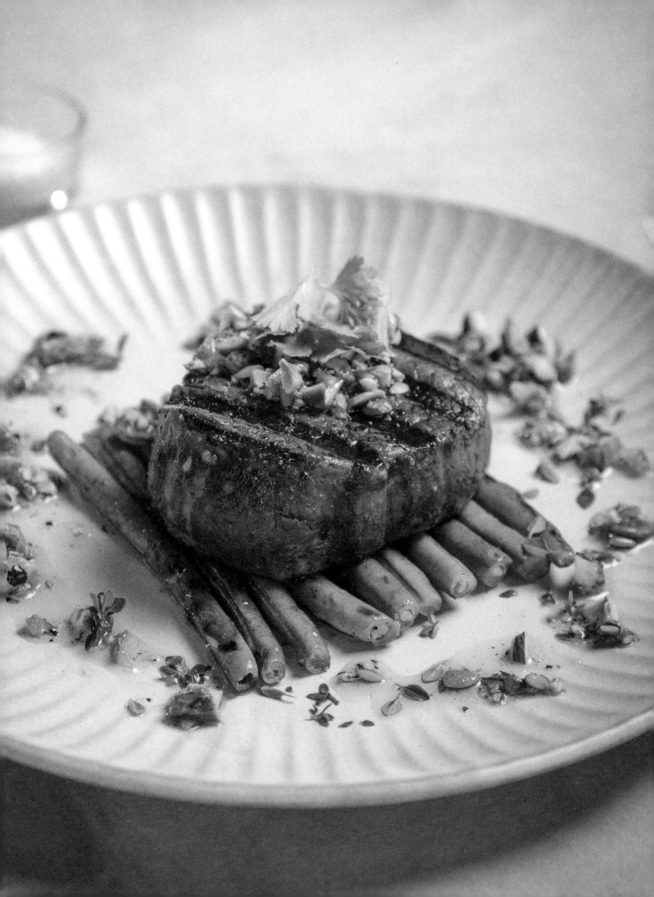

DF, GF, V, VG • **Vitamin C**

Quick Tomato, Walnut & Chickpea Stew

Serves 2–4
Prep: 5 minutes
Cook: 25 minutes

2 tbsp extra-virgin olive oil

1 onion, finely sliced

2 garlic cloves, crushed

1–2 tsp paprika, ground

1–2 tsp chilli flakes

4 Roma tomatoes, diced

400 g can chickpeas, drained
   and rinsed

1 jar tomato passata

sea salt and pepper, to taste

1 cup walnuts, finely chopped
   (can use a food processor)

1 bunch basil, chopped

Heat the extra-virgin olive oil in a frying pan, add the onion and cook for a few minutes before adding the garlic. Cook for an additional 2 minutes. Add the paprika and chilli flakes and fry off for 1 minute.

Add the diced fresh tomatoes and chickpeas and fry off for 4 minutes before adding the passata. Bring to a gentle boil and simmer for approximately 10 minutes, or until the mixture has thickened slightly.

Season to taste. Before taking off the heat, stir in the walnuts and basil.

—

As a post-workout meal, serve this stew on a bed of steamed quinoa for added protein and complex carbs.

DF, GF, V, VG • Zinc

Sweet Potato & Roasted Nut Quinoa Salad

Serves 6–8 (as a side)
Prep: 15 minutes
Cook: n/a

Dressing

⅓ cup tahini

2 tbsp extra-virgin olive oil/ water

1 tbsp lemon juice

2 tsp lemon zest

½ tbsp honey/maple syrup

1–2 garlic cloves, crushed

pinch cumin, ground

salt and pepper, to taste

Salad

2 cups kale leaves, finely chopped

1 tbsp extra-virgin olive oil

1½ cups sweet potato, peeled, cubed and steamed/roasted

2 cups quinoa, cooked

¾ cup fresh herbs (e.g. parsley, dill, coriander, thyme etc), chopped + extra to serve

¼ cup macadamia nuts, roughly chopped + extra to serve

¼ cup hazelnuts, skin removed, roughly chopped + extra to serve

¼ cup pine nuts + extra to serve

¼ cup dates, seeds removed, finely chopped

pinch salt and pepper

To make the dressing, whisk together all of the ingredients, adding more extra-virgin olive oil or water to thin, then season to taste.

To make the salad, add the kale leaves to a large bowl with the extra-virgin olive oil. Massage until the leaves slightly soften.

Add the remaining ingredients to the bowl and mix well.

Pour half of the dressing over the salad and mix.

Pour the remaining dressing over the top of the salad and sprinkle with the extra nuts and herbs.

—

Raw kale contains goitrogens, which in some individuals can affect iodine uptake and thyroid hormone production. If you have low thyroid function, cook kale before use or swap kale for rocket or fancy lettuce leaves.

GF, V • **Complex carbohydrates**

Nut, Quinoa & Herb Stuffed Sweet Potatoes

Makes 12
Prep: 20 minutes
Cook: 1 hour 15 minutes

6 small/medium sweet potatoes

1 tbsp extra-virgin olive oil

2 cups quinoa, cooked

¾ cup fresh herbs (e.g. parsley, dill, coriander, thyme etc), chopped

¼ cup macadamia nuts, roughly chopped

¼ cup hazelnuts, skin removed, roughly chopped

¼ cup pine nuts

¼ cup dates, seeds removed, finely chopped

1 tbsp lemon juice

2 tsp lemon zest

pinch salt and pepper

100–200 g goat's cheese, crumbled

Preheat the oven to 200°C. Line a baking tray with baking paper. Poke small holes in the sweet potatoes and drizzle them with the extra-virgin olive oil. Place them on the baking tray and bake for 40–60 minutes or until tender.

Meanwhile, in a bowl, combine the remaining ingredients excluding the goat's cheese.

Once the sweet potatoes are done, remove them from the oven and let cool slightly. Turn the oven down to 180°C.

Cut the sweet potatoes in half lengthways and scoop out half of the filling. Combine this filling with the quinoa herb mix.

Spoon the filling back into the sweet potato halves. Sprinkle with the goat's cheese and place back into the oven for 10–15 minutes to warm through.

Serve immediately.

—

Any leftover cooked grains can be used in place of quinoa.
For added veggies, try 1 cup quinoa and 1 cup cauliflower rice.

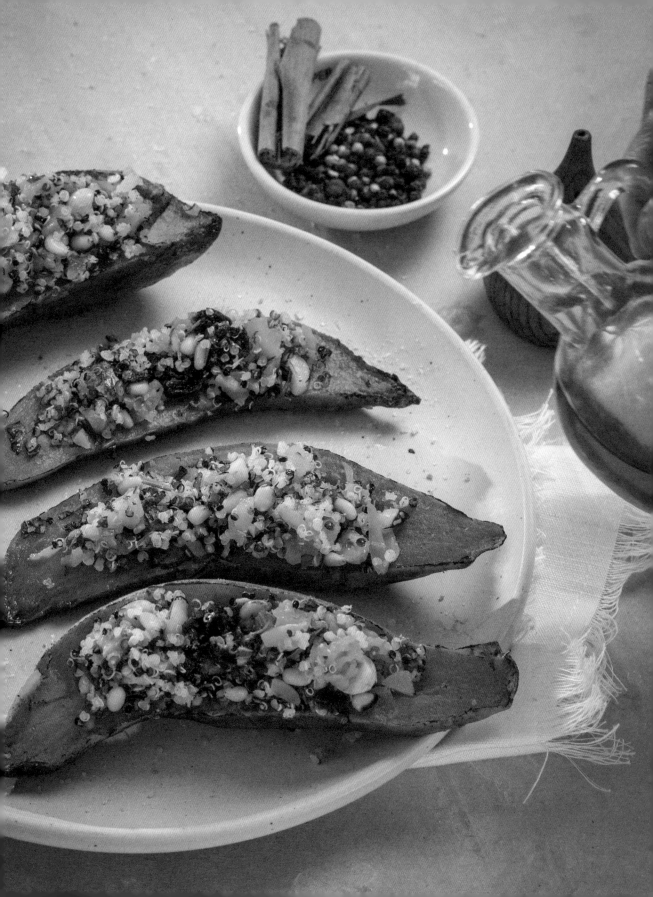

DF, V, VG • **Selenium**

Spaghetti with Mushroom & Tofu Balls

Serves 4
Prep: 10 minutes
Cook: 30 minutes

300 g hard tofu, crumbled

200 g button mushrooms, roughly chopped

1 onion, finely chopped

2 garlic cloves, crushed

½ bunch basil, finely chopped + extra to serve

1 carrot, peeled and grated

2 tbsp chia seeds + extra to serve

2–3 tsp sea salt and pepper

2–4 tbsp extra-virgin olive oil, for cooking

400 mL jar tomato pasta sauce

½–1 tsp lemon zest

½ packet wholemeal spaghetti, cooked according to packet directions

In a large bowl, combine the tofu, mushrooms, onion, garlic, basil, carrot, chia seeds, salt and pepper, and roll into small balls.

Heat the extra-virgin olive oil over a medium heat in a saucepan, then brown the tofu balls on each side. Pour the pasta sauce and lemon zest into the saucepan, bring to a gentle simmer and cook for 20–25 minutes until the meatballs are cooked through.

To serve, place cooked pasta into bowls and top with the meatballs and sauce. Finish with a few extra basil leaves and chia seeds.

—

If you have insulin resistance, swap wholemeal spaghetti for zucchini noodles or use half-and-half.

DF, GF, V, VG • **Vitamin C**

Roasted Cauliflower Salad with Spiced Almond Butter Dressing

Serves 6
Prep: 15 minutes
Cook: 30 minutes

Dressing

2 tbsp almond butter

dash tamari soy sauce, gluten-free

pinch chilli flakes

juice of 1 large orange + reserve zest to serve

water, to thin

Roasted Cauliflower Salad

2 tbsp extra-virgin olive oil

1 tbsp turmeric, ground

1 tsp cumin, ground

2 garlic cloves, crushed

salt and pepper

2–3 cups cauliflower, cut into florets

2–3 cups baby spinach leaves, to serve

fresh coriander leaves, chopped, to serve

Preheat the oven to 180°C.

To make the dressing, whisk together the almond butter, soy sauce and chilli flakes in a small bowl, adding the orange juice slowly and extra water as needed. Set aside.

In a small bowl, mix together the extra-virgin olive oil, turmeric, cumin, garlic, salt and pepper. Add the cauliflower and mix gently.

On a baking tray place the cauliflower mix, bake for 20-30 minutes or until golden on top and tender.

Remove from the oven. Serve on a bed of baby spinach leaves, and drizzle with the spiced almond butter dressing, coriander and orange zest.

—

For added protein and fibre, toss 1 cup cooked chickpeas or cannellini beans in with the cauliflower to be roasted.

DF • **Healthy fats**

Roasted Salmon & Eggplant Poke Plate

Serves 2–4
Prep: 30 minutes
Cook: 15 minutes

Roasted Salmon

1 tbsp soy sauce

1 tbsp mirin

1 tbsp light miso paste/bone
   broth paste

2 × 150 g fish fillets, salmon/
   white fish

Eggplant Poke

1 tbsp extra-virgin olive oil

¼ cup tahini

1 tbsp light miso paste

1 garlic clove, crushed

ice water

1 large eggplant, cut into
   rounds/4 baby eggplants,
   halved lengthways

1½ cups brown rice, cooked
   according to packet directions

Toppings

pickled ginger

1 avocado, seed and skin
   removed, diced

edamame

coriander, leaves picked

red chilli, seeds removed,
   finely sliced

spring onions, finely chopped

Combine the soy sauce, mirin, miso or bone broth paste in a bowl and mix well. Add the salmon fillets.

Preheat the oven to 180°C and line 2 baking trays with baking paper. On separate trays, place the salmon fillets and the eggplant drizzled with extra-virgin olive oil. Roast the eggplant for 15 minutes, flipping halfway. Roast the salmon for 10 minutes or until cooked to your liking, then gently flake apart into pieces.

To make the dressing, whisk together the tahini, miso paste and garlic and slowly add ice water until a smooth consistency is reached, then set aside.

To assemble the bowl, add the rice as the base, then layer the toppings and eggplant around the bowl and drizzle with the miso dressing.

—

Try adding edamame to this bowl as an added way to consume phytoestrogens. Bone broth powder can be purchased in the health section of major supermarkets, at health food stores or chemists. Miso paste is available from the Asian section of major supermarkets, Asian grocery stores or health food stores.

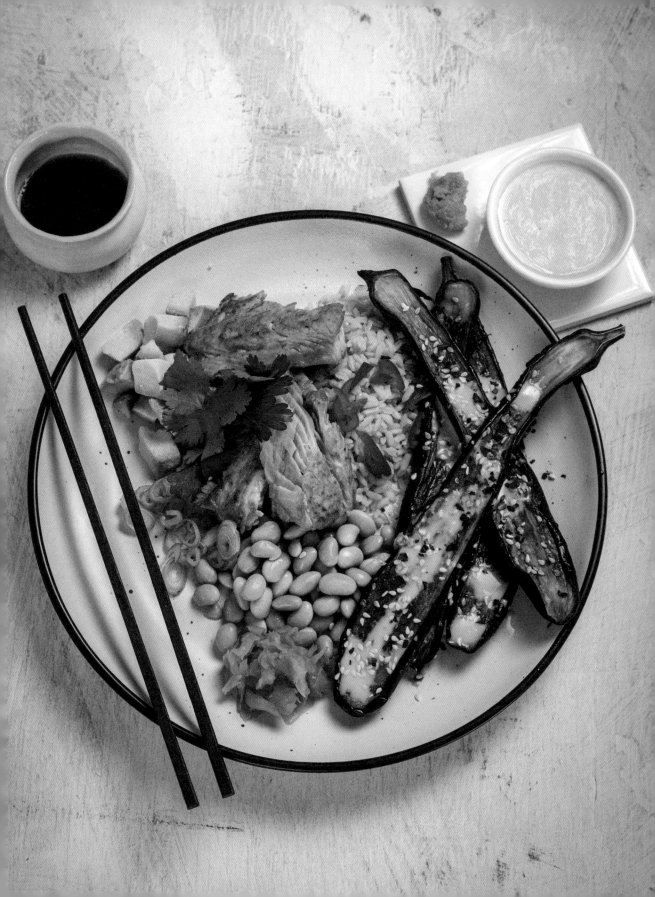

DF, GF • **B vitamins**

Chicken Thighs with Mushroom Sauce

Serves 4
Prep: 5 minutes
Cook: 40 minutes

1 tbsp extra-virgin olive oil

1 brown onion, thinly sliced

2 garlic cloves, crushed

2 cups mixed mushrooms,
   thinly sliced

1 tbsp lemon juice

1–2 tbsp lemon zest

200 mL bone broth (100 mL
   boiling water + 1 tsp bone
   broth powder) + extra if
   needed

2 tbsp fresh parsley, finely
   chopped

2 tbsp natural/coconut yoghurt

4 chicken thighs, trimmed and
   flattened

steamed greens of choice,
   to serve

For the sauce, heat the extra-virgin olive oil in a frying pan over a medium heat. Add the onion and sauté for 3 minutes. Add the garlic and cook for 1 minute. Add the mushrooms, lemon juice and lemon zest, then cook for a few minutes before adding the bone broth. Let simmer until the mushrooms are soft, then stir in the parsley. Take off the heat and stir through the yoghurt.

Meanwhile, pan-fry the chicken thighs on each side until cooked. Transfer to a plate, spoon over the mushroom sauce and serve with the steamed greens.

—

This recipe is ideal for men because mushrooms may assist to reduce aromatase enzyme activity and prevent the conversion of testosterone to oestrogen. Bone broth powder can be purchased in the health section of major supermarkets, at health food stores or chemists.

GF • **Protein**

Baked Seafood & Halloumi Parcels

Serves 2
Prep: 5–10 minutes
Cook: 25 minutes

1 zucchini, cut into batons

½ bunch basil, roughly chopped

4 Roma tomatoes, cut into rounds

2 tsp lemon zest

2 tbsp extra-virgin olive oil

sea salt and pepper, to taste

200 g mixed seafood

200 g halloumi, thickly sliced

lime, quartered, to serve

Preheat the oven to 180°C.

In a bowl, gently combine the zucchini, basil, tomatoes, lemon zest, olive oil, salt and pepper.

On a baking tray, place a large piece of baking paper and layer the vegetable mixture as a base. Place the fish and halloumi on top of the vegetables. Fold the baking paper in half and seal the bag airtight by twisting the edges together.

Bake in the oven for 15–25 minutes, or until cooked through.

Serve on a plate with a wedge of lime.

—

For a dairy-free version, omit halloumi and replace with ½ cup drained and rinsed cooked chickpeas or white beans.

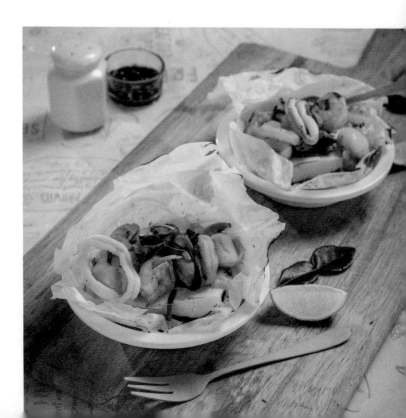

DF, GF, V, VG • **B vitamins**

Mushroom & Sweet Potato Shepherd's Pie

Serves 6
Prep: 10 minutes
Cook: 1 hour and 25 minutes

Filling

1 tbsp extra-virgin olive oil

1 leek, outer leaves removed, finely sliced

1 garlic clove, crushed

spice mix – 1 tsp each paprika, cumin, coriander seeds and turmeric, ground

500 g mixed mushrooms, roughly chopped

1 carrot, peeled and grated

400 g can crushed tomatoes

1 jar tomato passata

Topping

750 g sweet potato, peeled and chopped

1 tbsp extra-virgin olive oil

salt and pepper to taste

chia seeds

Preheat the oven to 180°C.

Heat the extra-virgin olive oil in a saucepan over a medium heat. Add the leek and cook for a few minutes or until soft, then add the garlic and cook for 2 minutes before adding the spice mix. Fry off for 1 minute.

Add the mushrooms to the pan and cook for 5 minutes until browned, before adding the carrot, tomatoes and passata. Bring to a gentle boil and simmer for 15–20 minutes until the veggies are tender. Spoon into an ovenproof dish or individual ramekins.

To make the topping, steam the sweet potato until tender, mash with the extra-virgin olive oil until smooth and season to taste.

Spoon the topping over the pie mixture, sprinkle with the chia seeds and bake for 20–25 minutes.

—

For added plant-based omega-3 fats, add ½ cup crushed walnuts to the mushroom mix.

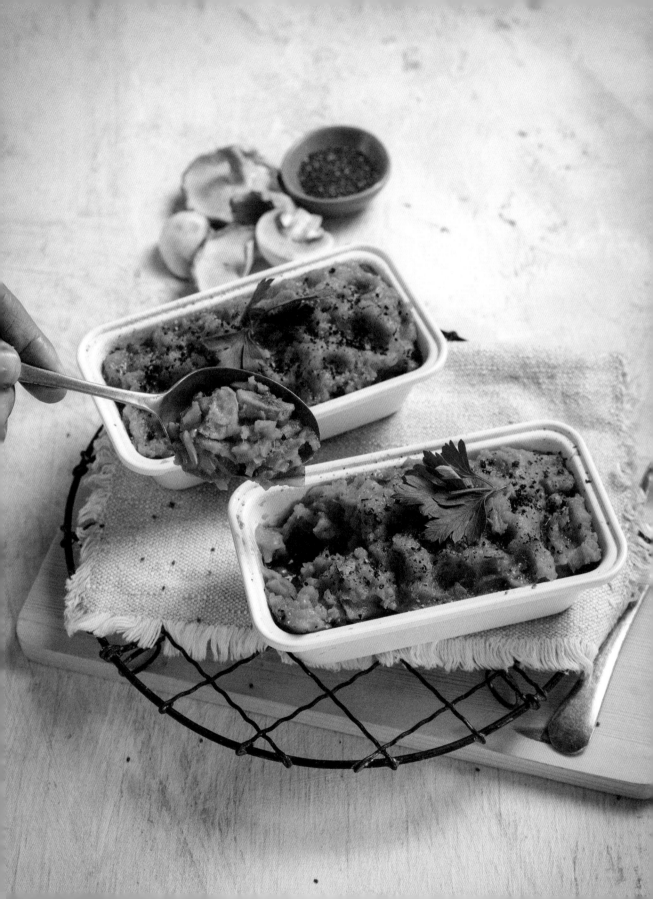

DF, GF • **Vitamin C**

Smoked Paprika Fish Tacos with Tomato Salsa

Serves 2–4
Prep: 20 minutes
Cook: 10–15 minutes

Salsa

1 avocado, seed and skin
  removed, diced

2 ripe tomatoes, finely diced

¼ cup red onion, finely diced

1 garlic clove, crushed

1–2 jalapeño chillies, seeds
  removed, finely sliced

1–2 fresh limes, reserve 1
  to serve

2 tbsp extra-virgin olive oil

sea salt and pepper, to taste

Fish

2 tbsp extra-virgin olive oil

300 g flathead/snapper fillets,
  cut into strips

¼ tsp cayenne pepper

¼ tsp paprika, ground

¼ tsp cumin, ground

¼ tsp turmeric, ground

sea salt and pepper, to taste

Assembly

4 corn tortillas/gluten-free
  wraps

1 cup cabbage slaw

For the salsa, combine the avocado, tomatoes, onion, garlic, jalapeño chilli, a squeeze of lime juice, extra-virgin olive oil, salt and pepper in a small bowl. Mix well and set aside to let the flavours develop.

Dust the fish with the cayenne pepper, paprika, cumin, turmeric, salt and pepper. Add the extra-virgin olive oil to the pan, before frying off the fish for a few minutes on each side, until golden.

Warm the corn tortillas in a microwave, pan or oven. Place a handful of slaw on each tortilla, then top with the fish, salsa, and finish with a squeeze of lime.

—

If making for other members of the family, you can serve in lettuce cups as a low carb option. This recipe is a good way for kids to get used to eating fish.

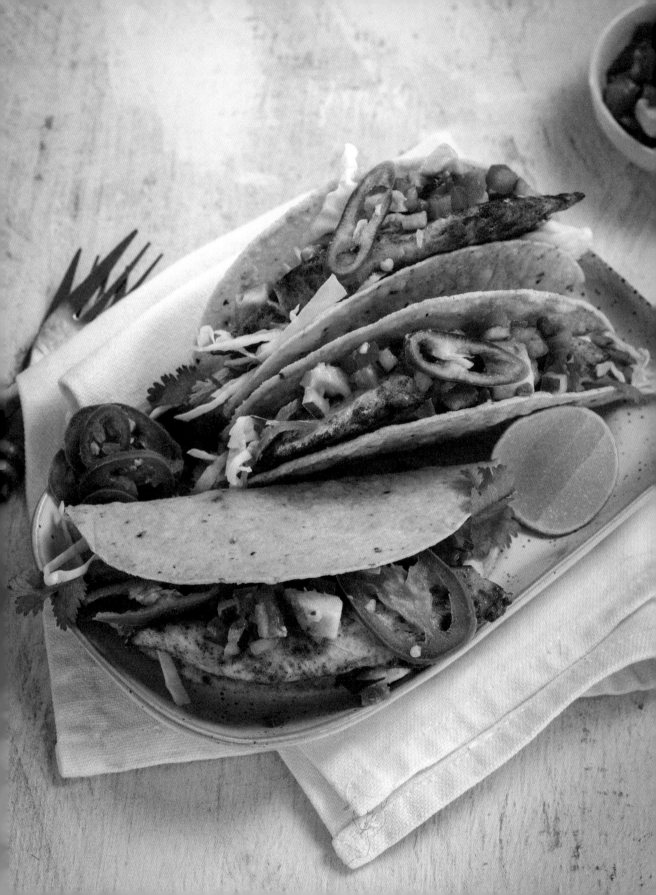

GF • Iron

Spring Lamb Cottage Pie with Cauliflower Top

Serves 6
Prep: 15 minutes
Cook: 1 hour and 20 minutes

To Serve

mixed lettuce leaves

extra-virgin olive oil

Pie Filling

1 tbsp extra-virgin olive oil

1 red onion, peeled and finely diced

2 garlic cloves, crushed

½ tsp paprika, ground

½ tsp cumin, ground

½ tsp coriander seeds, ground

500 g lamb mince

1 carrot, peeled and grated

4 fresh tomatoes, diced

½ bunch basil, finely chopped

500 g jar tomato passata

salt and pepper, to taste

Topping

1 small head cauliflower, leaves removed, cut into florets

⅓ cup cow's/soy/almond milk + extra if needed

salt and pepper, to taste

2 Roma tomatoes, sliced into thin rounds

⅓ cup parmesan cheese, grated

pinch cayenne pepper

Preheat the oven to 180°C.

Heat the extra-virgin olive oil in a saucepan over a medium heat, then add the onion and cook for a few minutes until soft. Add the garlic, then cook for 2 minutes before adding the paprika, cumin and coriander seeds. Fry off for 1 minute.

Add the lamb mince to the pan and cook for 5 minutes until browned before adding the carrot, tomatoes, basil and passata.

Bring to a gentle boil and simmer for 15–20 minutes until the mince is cooked, season to taste. Spoon the mixture into 6 individual ramekins.

To make the topping, steam the cauliflower until tender. Add to a food processor or blender and start blending while adding the milk until a smooth consistency is reached, then season to taste.

Top each ramekin of mince mixture with the sliced tomato, cauliflower mash, parmesan cheese and a sprinkle of cayenne pepper.

Bake in the oven for 20–30 minutes until the top has started to lightly brown.

Remove from the oven and serve on a plate with the mixed lettuce leaves drizzled with extra-virgin olive oil.

—

For a vegetarian version, replace lamb mince with 1 cup cooked lentils and 2 cups raw diced mushrooms. To get kids involved with this recipe, ask them to decorate the top of the pie with the toppings.

DF, GF • Iron

Sumac Lamb Fillets with Cauliflower Tabouli & Coconut Tzatziki

Serves 2
Prep: 20 minutes (+ 4 hours or
* overnight marinating time)*
Cook: 35 minutes

Lamb

200 g lamb backstrap/fillet

1 tbsp extra-virgin olive oil

¼ tsp sumac, ground/lemon
  zest

1 tbsp lemon juice

½ tsp lemon zest

salt and pepper

Cauliflower Tabouli

150 g cauliflower, cut into florets

sea salt and pepper

¼ tsp sumac, ground/lemon
  zest

1½ tbsp extra-virgin olive oil

1 cup kale, finely chopped

2 small Roma tomatoes, seeds
  removed, finely diced

¼ bunch parsley, finely chopped

3 tbsp pine nuts

1 tbsp extra-virgin olive oil

1 tbsp lemon juice

Coconut Yoghurt Tzatziki

¼ cup coconut yoghurt

1 small cucumber, grated and
  moisture squeezed out

1 tbsp lemon juice

1 garlic clove, crushed

sea salt, to taste

Place all of the lamb ingredients into a glass bowl and marinate for 4 hours, or overnight (optional).

Preheat the oven to 180°C.

Line a baking tray with baking paper, add the cauliflower and sprinkle with the salt, pepper, sumac and extra-virgin olive oil. Roast for 30 minutes or until tender. Remove from the heat and let cool slightly.

Heat a pan over a medium-high heat, add the lamb and cook on each side for a few minutes, until cooked to your liking. Remove from the heat and let stand for 10 minutes before slicing.

Meanwhile, in a large bowl, add the cauliflower mix, kale, tomatoes, pine nuts and parsley, mixing well. Drizzle with the extra-virgin olive oil and lemon juice and season to taste, then set aside.

To make the coconut yoghurt tzatziki, mix together all of the ingredients in a small bowl.

Pile the salad on a plate, top with the lamb and finish with a dollop of coconut yoghurt tzatziki.

—

For added health benefits, try adding dried lemon myrtle to the sumac marinade for the lamb. Lemon myrtle contains folate, vitamins A and E, zinc and magnesium.

V • **Vitamin C**

Spelt Gnocchi with Rich Tomato Sauce

Serves 2
Prep: 15–20 minutes
Cook: 25 minutes

1 cup baby spinach leaves, very finely chopped

250 g fresh ricotta

1 large egg, lightly beaten

pinch nutmeg, freshly grated

½ cup parmesan cheese, freshly grated + extra to serve

¾ cup spelt flour + extra for flouring work surface

¼ cup extra-virgin olive oil

1 punnet Perino/grape tomatoes, roughly chopped

zest of ½ lemon + extra to serve

1 tsp fresh parsley, roughly chopped + extra to serve

½ tsp chilli flakes

1–2 garlic cloves, finely chopped

1–2 tsp sea salt and pepper

Bring a large saucepan of water to a boil with a pinch of salt.

In a large bowl, combine the spinach with the ricotta, egg, nutmeg and parmesan and mix to combine. Add the spelt flour and combine into dough. Place the gnocchi dough onto a lightly floured work surface and gently knead until smooth.

Cut into small pieces and gently add to the boiling water. Cook for approximately 5 minutes.

In a saucepan, add the extra-virgin olive oil, tomatoes, lemon zest, parsley, chilli flakes, garlic, salt and pepper and cook for 10 minutes.

Carefully transfer the gnocchi to the tomato sauce and stir lightly to heat through. Spoon into shallow bowls and serve with additional lemon zest and parsley on top.

—

If your kids need extra protein, try blending some brown lentils into the tomato sauce before adding the gnocchi to the pan.

V • Protein

Chickpea, Tofu & Spinach Pasta

Serves 4–6
Prep: 10 minutes
Cook: 20 minutes

250–300 g spelt pasta,
spirals/penne

3 tbsp extra-virgin olive oil

200 g hard organic tofu,
crumbled

2 garlic cloves, crushed

1 red chilli, seeds removed,
finely sliced

1 x 400 g tin chickpeas, drained
and rinsed

½–1 cup vegetable stock/
miso stock (1 tbsp miso paste
+ 1 cup warm water)

60 g baby spinach leaves

¼ cup flat leaf parsley, chopped

½ cup feta cheese, crumbled

salt and pepper, to taste

Cook the pasta as per the packet directions, then drain.

Heat the extra-virgin olive oil in a pan over a medium heat. Add the tofu and cook by breaking up with a spoon until opaque, approximately 4 minutes.

Add the garlic and chilli to the pan and cook for 1 minute.

Next add the chickpeas and vegetable stock and cook for 3 minutes. Combine well before stirring in the spinach and parsley. Add the pasta, reduce heat to low and cook for 2 minutes.

Just before taking off the heat, fold through the feta cheese and season to taste.

—

Using spelt pasta is a good way to boost the overall protein content of this meal. Legume pasta can also be used.

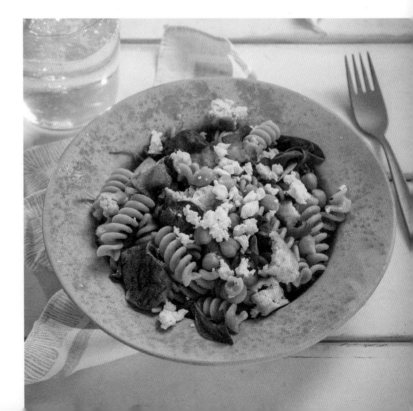

DF, GF • **Vitamin C**

Whole Baked Trout Side with Native Herb, Pink Grapefruit & Aioli

Serves 10
Prep: 15 minutes
Cook: 20 minutes

Citrus Aioli

2 egg yolks, at room
  temperature

1–2 tbsp lemon juice/apple
  cider vinegar

1–2 garlic cloves, crushed

350 mL extra-virgin olive oil

Whole Baked Trout

1 kg approximately side of trout/
  salmon, skin on

native herbs – 2 tsp lemon
  myrtle, ground and 1–2 tsp
  Kakadu plum/lemongrass

2 garlic cloves, crushed

sea salt and pepper, to taste

2–4 tbsp extra-virgin olive oil

1 large/2 small blood oranges/
  pink grapefruits/oranges,
  thinly sliced

½ bunch parsley/coriander,
  stalks removed + extra to
  serve

Preheat the oven to 180°C.

To make the aioli, place the egg yolks, lemon and garlic into a food processor or hand whisk and blend until smooth. With the motor running or while whisking, slowly add the extra-virgin olive oil until the mixture is emulsified.

Place the fish on a large sheet of baking paper (or alfoil). Rub the fish with the native herbs, garlic, salt, pepper and extra-virgin olive oil.

Along 1 side of the fish, lay the sliced orange or grapefruit and parsley. Place the fish in the oven for approximately 20 minutes, or until cooked to your liking.

Remove from the oven and cut into portions to serve, topped with the fresh herbs and aioli on the side.

—

For a twist on the aioli, try using macadamia nut oil in place of extra-virgin olive oil.

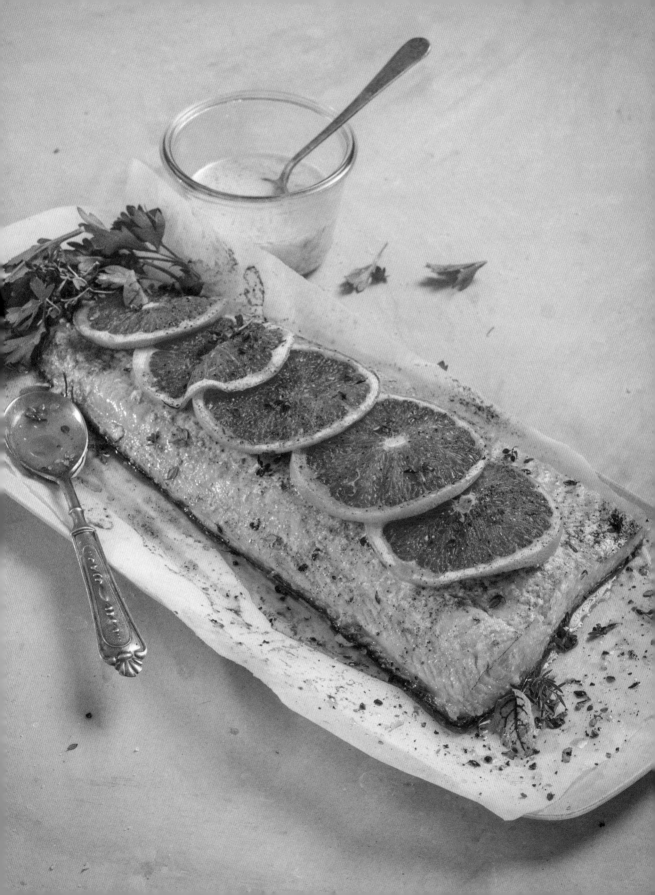

DF, GF, V, VG • Zinc

Whole Spiced Roasted Cauliflower with Roasted Capsicum Hummus

Serves 4
Prep: 10 minutes
Cook: 1 hour

Topping

2 tbsp fresh herbs, chopped

2 tbsp nuts/seeds, chopped

2 tbsp pomegranate seeds, optional

2 tbsp extra-virgin olive oil

Roasted Cauliflower

½ tsp cumin, ground

½ tsp ginger, ground

¼ tsp paprika, ground

¼ tsp cinnamon, ground

¼ tsp turmeric, ground

¼ tsp coriander seeds, ground

¼ tsp salt

¼ tsp black pepper

3 tbsp extra-virgin olive oil

1 medium head of cauliflower, leaves trimmed

Roasted Capsicum Hummus

1 red capsicum

400 g can chickpeas, drained and rinsed

½ cup tahini

2 tbsp lemon juice

¼ tsp cayenne pepper, optional

2 garlic cloves, crushed

2 tbsp extra-virgin olive oil

sea salt and pepper, to taste

Preheat the oven to 180°C and line 2 baking trays with baking paper.

To make the cauliflower, in a small bowl mix together all of the spices. Add the extra-virgin olive oil and mix until a paste forms.

Rub the cauliflower with the spice paste and coat well, then place on a baking tray.

Place the capsicum on the second tray.

Put both trays into the oven and cook for 30–60 minutes until both the cauliflower and capsicum are tender and well roasted. The capsicum will cook faster, so remove it first.

Once removed from the oven, set the cauliflower aside and remove the skin and seeds from the capsicum before cutting into strips.

In a food processor or blender, add the capsicum, chickpeas, tahini, lemon juice, cayenne pepper, garlic and extra-virgin olive oil and blend until smooth, adding more oil if needed. Season to taste.

Spoon the hummus onto the base of a serving dish, top with the roasted cauliflower and finish with the fresh herbs, nuts, seeds, pomegranate seeds and a drizzle of extra-virgin olive oil.

—

If sensitive to spicy food, omit cayenne pepper from the roasted capsicum hummus and replace with paprika.

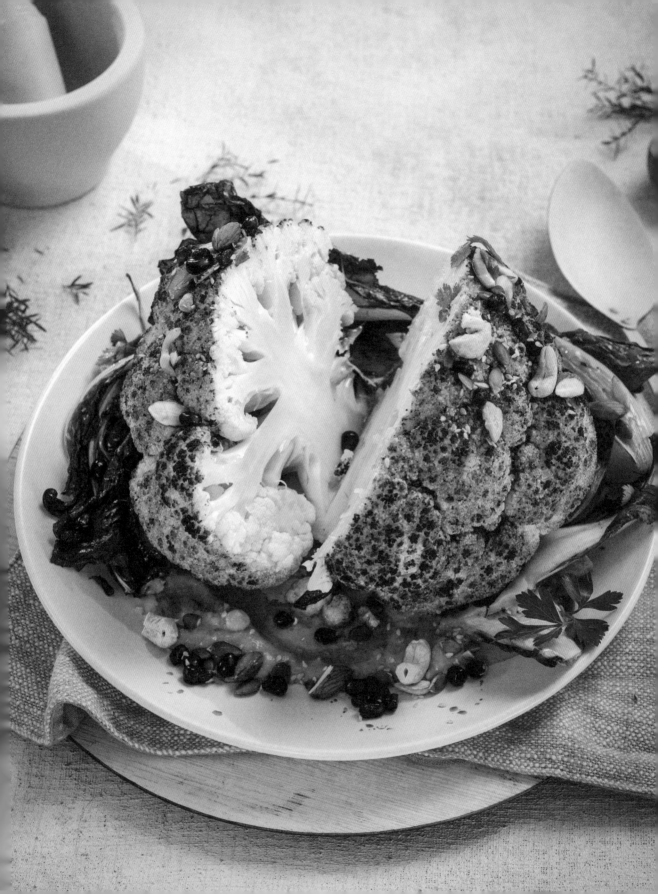

Sauces
and Sides

DF, GF, V, VG • **Antioxidants**

Fermented Beetroot Relish

Serves 2-4
Prep: 15 minutes
Cook: n/a

½ cup fermented beetroot

¼ cup red apple, diced

1 small Spanish onion, finely chopped

1 tbsp macadamia nuts, toasted and chopped

½ tbsp pomegranate molasses

½ tbsp extra-virgin olive oil

pinch salt and pepper

Roughly dice the fermented beetroot.

In a small bowl, add all of the ingredients. Mix well.

—

This relish is a delicious way to add a little bit of sweetness to savoury dishes. Pomegranate molasses is available from gourmet delis or the international section of major supermarkets.

DF, GF, V • **Antioxidants**

Garlic Citrus Aioli

Serves 4–6
Prep: 20 minutes
Cook: n/a

2 egg yolks, at room temperature

1–2 tbsp lemon juice/apple cider vinegar

1–2 garlic cloves, crushed

350 mL extra-virgin olive oil

To make the aioli, place the egg yolks, lemon juice and garlic into a food processor or hand whisk and blend until smooth. With the motor running or while whisking, slowly add the extra-virgin olive oil until the mixture is emulsified.

—

For a richer flavour, use roasted garlic instead of fresh.

DF, GF, V, VG • **Antioxidants**

Fermented Cumin Beetroot Salsa

Serves 4–5
Prep: 30 minutes (+ fermenting time)
Cook: n/a

500 g mix purple and golden beetroots, scrubbed, tops and ends removed

½ tsp mustard seeds

½ tsp celery salt

½ tsp cumin seeds

peel of 1 orange

½ tbsp salt

300 mL water

Sterilise a 500 mL jar, then dry. Thinly slice the beetroot using a mandolin, or dice. Place the beetroot, mustard seeds, celery salt, cumin seeds and orange peel into the jar.

In a small bowl, mix together the water and salt and pour into the jar, enough to cover the beetroot.

Place a lid on the jar. Label with today's date.

Let the jar sit at room temperature for approximately 1 week. Open and close the jar every few days to let any built-up air to be released.

Move to the fridge, once happy with the flavour.

—

This salsa is a delicious way to add fibre to meals.

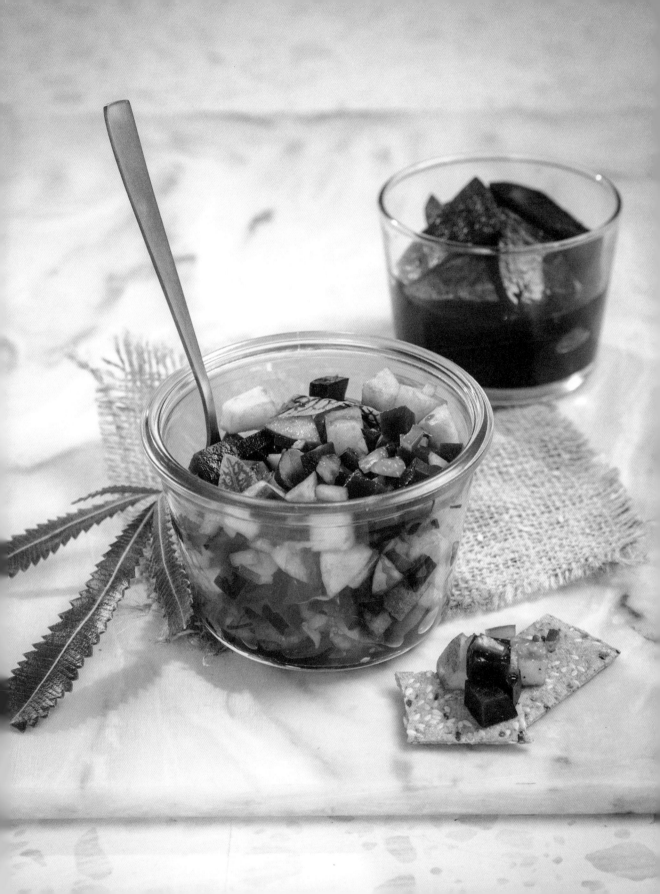

GF, V • Vitamin C

Roasted Cauliflower & Feta Salad with Green Tahini Dressing

Serves 2
Prep: 10 minutes
Cook: 30 minutes

Salad

1 small head cauliflower, cut into florets

1 small red onion, peeled and sliced

5 mL extra-virgin olive oil

salt and pepper, to taste

1 cup kale leaves, roughly chopped

1 small avocado, seed and skin removed, diced

30 g feta cheese, crumbled + reserve some to serve

75 g grape tomatoes, quartered

Green Tahini Dressing

15 g cashews, soaked overnight and drained

1 tbsp tahini

½ small bunch parsley, chopped

1 tbsp lemon juice/apple cider vinegar

1 garlic clove, crushed

salt and pepper

Preheat the oven to 180°C.

Line a baking tray with baking paper. Add the cauliflower and onion to the tray, drizzle with the extra-virgin olive oil, salt and pepper, and bake for 30 minutes until tender and crispy. Remove from the heat and let cool.

To make the dressing, add all of the ingredients to a blender and blend until smooth, adding boiling water to thin, if needed. Set aside.

In a large bowl, add the kale and half of the dressing. Massage the kale leaves until tender. Add the baked cauliflower and onion, avocado, half of the feta and tomatoes, and gently combine. Drizzle with more dressing and sprinkle with the remaining feta and serve.

—

Swap kale for rocket if you have hypothyroidism and are sensitive to goitrogens.

GF, V • **Prebiotics**

Asparagus with Feta & Pepita Salsa

Serves 2 or 4 (as a side)
Prep: 10 minutes
Cook: 5 minutes

100 g feta/goat's cheese, crumbled

2 tbsp green olives, finely chopped

2 tbsp basil leaves, finely chopped

1 tbsp lemon juice

1–2 tbsp extra-virgin olive oil/ melted butter

¼ cup pepitas/pumpkin seeds/ pine nuts

1 bunch asparagus, ends trimmed

In a bowl, combine the cheese, olives, basil, lemon juice, a drizzle of extra-virgin olive oil and pepitas. Set aside.

In a small steamer, boil water and steam the asparagus for a few minutes until still firm, then remove and place in a bowl full of ice water for a few minutes. Remove, drain and pat dry.

In a small bowl, drizzle the asparagus with the extra-virgin olive oil and combine well. Place the asparagus on a plate and top with the cheese and pepitas mix.

—

Asparagus contains inulin, a prebiotic fibre, and therefore helps to produce short-chain fatty acids (SCFAs), which play an important role in gut health.

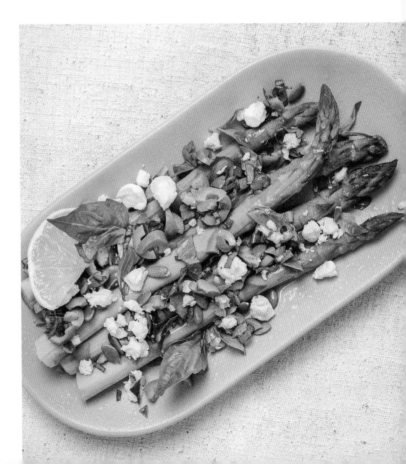

DF, GF • Iodine

Japanese Rice Cones

Makes 8–10 cones
Prep: 10 minutes
  (+ 30 minutes cooling time)
Cook: 30 minutes

Rice Cones

2 cups short-grain brown rice

3 cups water

1 cup carrot, grated

½ bunch chives, finely chopped

1 tbsp tamari soy sauce,
  gluten-free

4–8 nori sheets

½ cup mix black and white
  sesame seeds

Fillings

avocado, cut into 2–3 cm cubes,
  drizzled with lemon juice

tofu, cut into 2–3 cm cubes,
  cooked

2 tsp mix salmon mashed with
  avocado

Place the rice and water in a saucepan, then cover with a lid and bring to the boil. Turn the heat down and simmer over a low heat for approximately 30 minutes. Once the rice has absorbed all of the water, remove from heat and let rest until cooled.

Transfer the rice to a large bowl, then add the carrot, chives and soy sauce. Mix well.

Take a nori sheet and roll into a cone shape, then slightly wet the end and seal. Spoon the fillings into the cone and work the rice around the fillings until you have a ball. Sprinkle with the sesame seeds, place on a baking tray, and repeat the process until all the rice has been used. Cover and refrigerate for 30 minutes.

—

If your kids enjoy these cones, roasted nori sheets also make a yummy snack – rich in iodine, important for brain health. These are a great make-at-home twist on sushi that kids can get involved in.

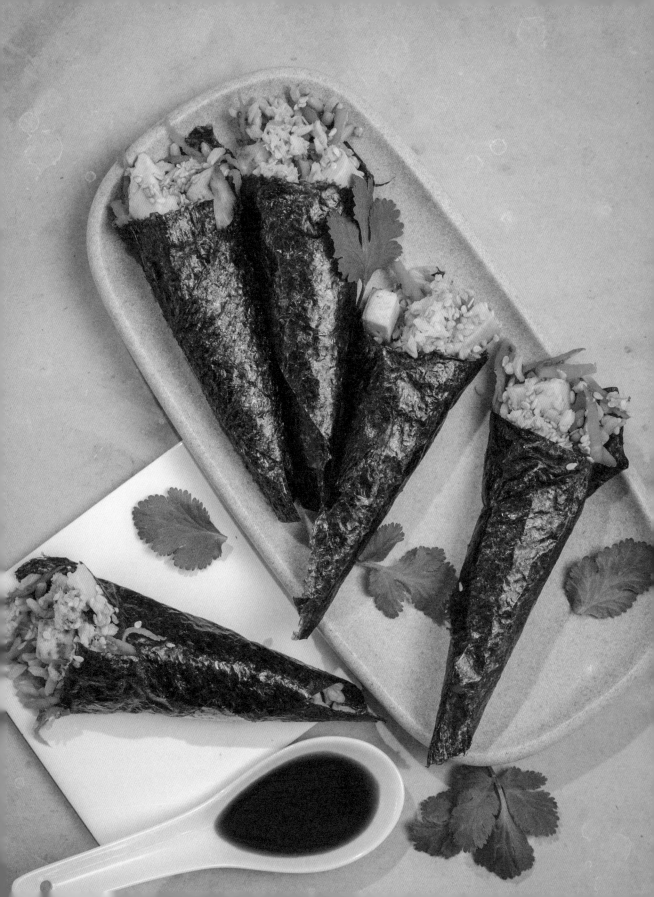

GF, V • **Vitamin C**

Spice Roasted Carrot & Smoked Almond Herb Salad

Serves 4–6 (as a side)
Prep: 15 minutes
Cook: 30 minutes

500 g carrots, peeled and thickly sliced diagonally

3 tbsp extra-virgin olive oil

½ tbsp sea salt

½ tbsp cumin, ground

½ tbsp coriander seeds, ground

½ tbsp smoked paprika, ground

½ cup smoked almonds, skin on and roughly chopped

100 g feta/goat's cheese, crumbled, to serve

½ cup fresh coriander leaves, chopped, to serve

½ cup fresh mint leaves, roughly chopped, to serve

½ cup fresh parsley leaves, chopped, to serve

squeeze lemon/orange juice, to serve

Preheat the oven to 180–200°C.

Place the carrots in a baking dish, drizzle with the extra-virgin olive oil and add the sea salt, cumin, coriander seeds and smoked paprika. Toss well.

Roast until tender for 15–20 minutes, then add the almonds and further roast for 10 minutes, or until golden brown.

Take out of the oven, place on a serving dish and top with the cheese, coriander, mint, parsley and a squeeze of juice.

—

To support liver detox, add raw beetroot to the baking dish and roast until soft.

DF, GF, V, VG • **Vitamin C**

Chunky Spirulina Guacamole

Serves 2–4
Prep: 5 minutes
Cook: n/a

1 large ripe avocado, seed and
  skin removed, diced

1 tbsp lime juice

1 garlic clove, crushed

½ tsp spirulina powder

1 tbsp extra-virgin olive oil

2 tbsp coriander, chopped

1 red chilli, seeds removed,
  finely sliced, optional

1 tomato, chopped

½ bunch spring onions, finely
  chopped

salt and pepper, to taste

Place all of the ingredients in a bowl and mash until desired
consistency is reached.

—

*Crumbled feta or goat's cheese is also a yummy addition to this
guacamole. Spirulina can be purchased in the health section of
major supermarkets, at health food stores or chemists.*

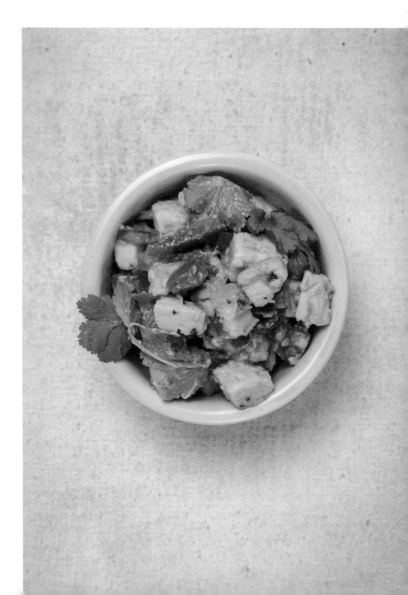

DF, GF, V, VG • **Antioxidants**

Roasted Beetroot & Hemp Seed Hummus

Serves 4–6
Prep: 15 minutes
Cook: 30 minutes

½ large beetroot, cubed

2 tbsp extra-virgin olive oil
  + extra to thin and to drizzle

salt and pepper, to taste

1 tbsp tahini

1 tbsp hemp seeds

1 tbsp lemon juice

½ tsp lemon zest

½ tsp cumin, ground

1 garlic clove, crushed

parsley, chopped, to serve

Preheat the oven to 200°C. In a baking dish, place the beetroot, extra-virgin olive oil, and a little salt and pepper. Bake for 20–30 minutes until tender.

Combine the beetroot, tahini, hemp, lemon, cumin and garlic in a food processor until well combined, adding more oil until desired consistency is reached.

Top with the parsley and a drizzle of the extra-virgin olive oil.

—

For added antioxidant support, try adding 1–2 tsp beetroot powder before blending.

DF, GF, V, VG • Fibre

Tofu Avocado Mayo

Serves 6–8
Prep: 5 minutes
Cook: n/a

1 medium avocado, seed and
   skin removed

150 g silken tofu, drained

1 tbsp lime juice

½ tsp honey/maple syrup

2 tbsp hemp seeds

2–3 tsp miso paste, gluten-free

Combine all of the ingredients in a blender or food processor
and blend until smooth. Adjust seasoning to suit.

—

*This mayo is a great way to sneak in protein, especially if feeding
kids! Miso paste is available from the Asian section of major
supermarkets, Asian grocery stores or health food stores.*

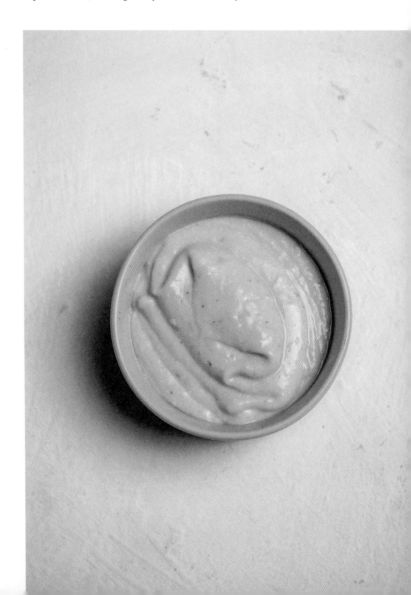

DF, GF, V, VG • **Iron**

Quick Carrot Hummus

Serves 4–6
Prep: 15 minutes
Cook: n/a

400 g can chickpeas, drained

2 tbsp tahini

1 tbsp lemon juice

pinch turmeric, ground

1 cup carrot, grated

2–4 tbsp extra-virgin olive oil/
water

black sesame seeds, to serve

Combine all of the ingredients except the black sesame seeds in a high-powered blender or food processor and process until combined. Add additional extra-virgin olive oil or water until a smooth consistency is reached.

Pack in a small container and sprinkle with the black sesame seeds. Serve with vegetable sticks or seed crackers.

—

This hummus also works well as a wrap or sandwich spread in the lunchbox.

DF, GF, V, VG • **Fibre**

Roasted Turmeric, Walnut & Sweet Potato Dip

Serves 4–6
Prep: 10 minutes
Cook: n/a

1–1½ cups sweet potato, steamed/roasted

2–4 tbsp olive oil

¼ cup walnuts, roasted + extra to serve

½ tbsp lemon juice/orange juice

½ tsp turmeric, ground/freshly grated

½ tsp cumin, ground

salt and pepper, to taste

Add all of the ingredients to a food processor and blitz until well combined and smooth, adding more olive oil or water until desired consistency is reached. Season to taste, then top with the extra walnuts.

—

This dip also works well as a mash – add to a pan with a splash of stock to thin out and warm up.

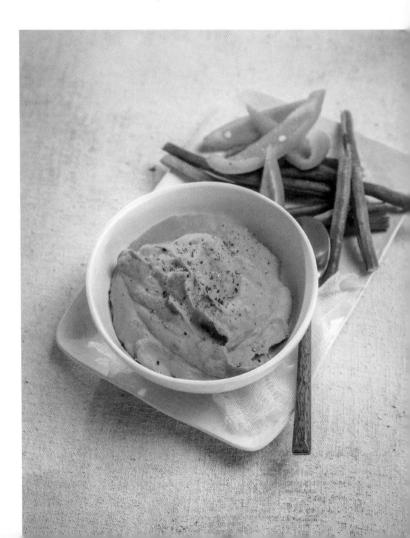

DF, GF, V • **Healthy fats**

Macadamia Nut Pâté

Serves 6–8
Prep: 5 minutes
Cook: 15 minutes

2 tbsp extra-virgin olive oil

1 onion, chopped

1 celery stick, chopped

1 garlic clove, chopped

100 g button mushrooms,
  finely sliced

50 g macadamia nuts, chopped

175 g cashews, finely ground

1 egg, beaten

good pinch paprika, ground

good pinch dried thyme

salt and black pepper, to taste

4 wholemeal pita breads
  (gluten-free if required), cut
  into triangles

In a large frying pan, heat the extra-virgin olive oil and add the onion, celery, garlic and mushroom. Cook for 5–10 minutes until lightly golden brown. Remove from the heat and stir in the macadamia nuts, ground cashews, egg, paprika and thyme. Add the salt and pepper to taste. Spoon into a ramekin and allow to cool.

Preheat the oven to 200°C. Place the pita bread on a baking tray and toast until brown. Serve the pâté with the pita bread on the side.

—

To boost the healthy fat intake of your meals, try using this pâté as a spread for sandwiches, toast or wraps.

DF, GF, V, VG • **Healthy fats**

Macadamia Hummus

Serves 6
Prep: 5 minutes
Cook: n/a

Hummus

100 g raw macadamia nuts,
   soaked overnight and drained

1–2 garlic cloves, crushed

50 g tahini

40 mL extra-virgin olive oil

2–4 tbsp warm water

pinch chilli flakes

pinch cumin, ground

salt and pepper, to taste

To Serve

cucumber, celery, capsicum,
   broccoli crudités

In a blender, add all of the hummus ingredients and blend until the mixture becomes smooth. Season to taste.

Serve the hummus in a bowl alongside the vegetables.

—

Turmeric is a lovely addition for added anti-inflammatory benefits.

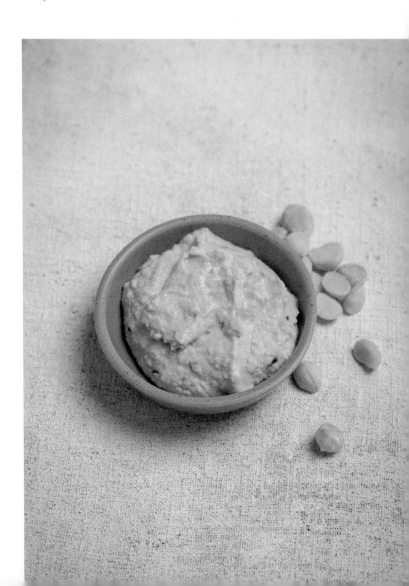

DF, GF, V, VG • **Fibre**

Seed Crackers with Fresh Tomato Salsa

Serves 8–10
Prep: 25 minutes
Cook: 15–20 minutes

Fresh Salsa

2 large Roma tomatoes, finely diced

½ bunch spring onions, outer leaves removed, finely diced

1 long red chilli, seeds removed, finely diced

1 cucumber, finely diced

¼ bunch coriander, finely diced

1 tbsp extra-virgin olive oil

1 tbsp lime juice

salt and pepper, to taste

1–2 garlic cloves, crushed

Seed Crackers

¼ cup flaxseeds

2 tbsp chia seeds

1 tbsp hemp seeds

1 tbsp sesame seeds

⅓ cup pumpkin seeds

⅓ cup sunflower seeds

1 tsp psyllium husk

pinch salt

1 cup boiling water + extra if needed

To make the salsa, combine all of the ingredients in a small bowl and adjust the seasoning to suit. Set aside in the fridge.

Preheat the oven to 160°C and line a baking tray with non-stick baking paper.

In a large bowl, combine all of the cracker ingredients, except the water. Add a small amount of water at a time until the mixture comes together. Let stand for 10 minutes.

Spread the seed mixture in a thin layer over the baking paper and score cracker shapes in the mixture.

Place in the oven for 15 minutes or until lightly golden. Let cool on the tray and break into crackers.

Serve the seed crackers with the salsa.

—

These seed crackers are rich in healthy fats and fibre, making them a great mid-afternoon choice to prevent snacking and grazing all the way to dinnertime!

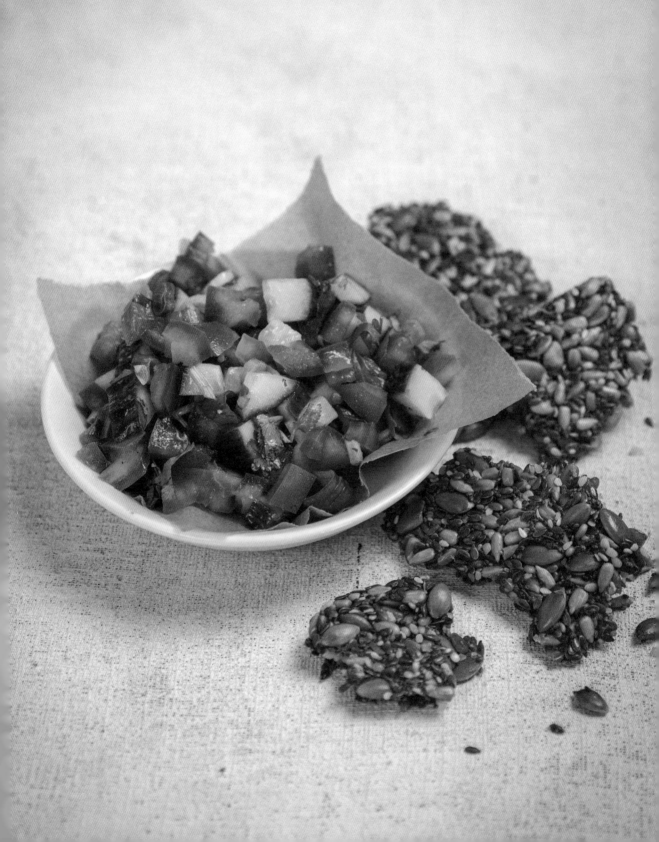

GF, V • **Vitamin C**

Turmeric & Tahini Cauliflower 'Rice' Salad

Serves 4
Prep: 15 minutes
Cook: 15 minutes

Tahini Dressing

1 garlic clove, crushed

1 tbsp lemon juice/½ tbsp
apple cider vinegar

1 tbsp tahini

½ tsp honey

½ tsp cumin, ground

¼ cup extra-virgin olive oil

salt and pepper to taste

Salad

2 cups cauliflower, cut into florets

1 tbsp extra-virgin olive oil/
coconut oil

1 leek, outer leaves removed,
finely sliced

2 tsp turmeric, powder/freshly
grated

handful baby spinach leaves

handful fresh coriander leaves,
chopped + reserve some to
serve

½ punnet grape tomatoes,
halved

100 g goat's cheese, crumbled

½ cup pomegranate seeds/
cranberries + extra to serve

¼ cup pistachios

To make the dressing, whisk all of the ingredients together in a small bowl, then set aside.

Place the cauliflower florets in a food processor and pulse until a 'rice' consistency forms, then set aside.

Heat the oil over a medium heat in a frying pan, add the leek and sauté for a few minutes until soft, then add the turmeric and fry off for 1 minute.

Add the cauliflower rice to the pan and gently stir-fry until golden from the turmeric. Add the spinach and half of the coriander leaves, then take off the heat once lightly wilted.

In a bowl, combine the cauliflower mix, tomatoes, half of the goat's cheese, pomegranate seeds and pistachios. Crumble remaining goat's cheese over the top of the salad before drizzling over the dressing.

Finish with a sprinkle of the pomegranate seeds and fresh coriander.

—

As an alternative, use 1 cup cauliflower and 1 cup broccoli.

DF, GF, V, VG • **Zinc**

Nut Salsa Verde

Serves 4
  (save extra in a jar and
  refrigerate)
Prep: 15 minutes
Cook: n/a

To make the nut salsa verde, combine all of the ingredients in a bowl and mix well. Set aside in the fridge.

—

Hazelnuts also work well as an alternative to pistachios.

2 tbsp pumpkin seeds, crushed

2 tbsp pistachios, crushed

½ cup fresh coriander, stems removed, finely chopped

1 tbsp lemon zest

1 garlic clove, crushed

1 green chilli, seeds removed, thinly sliced

2 tbsp extra-virgin olive oil

salt and pepper, to taste

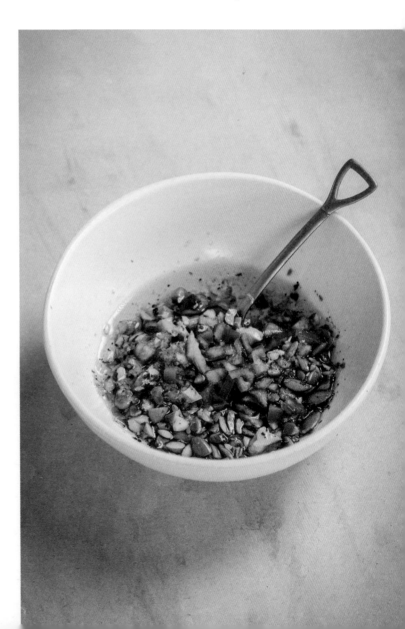

GF, V • **Vitamin C**

Orange, Goat's Cheese, Almond & Quinoa Salad

Serves 4 (as a side)
Prep: 15 minutes
Cook: 20 minutes

Salad

½ cup quinoa, raw

1 cup water

1 medium beetroot, peeled, roasted and diced

1 orange, peeled and segmented

½ bunch coriander, finely chopped

½ cup dry roasted almonds, chopped

50 g feta/goat's cheese, crumbled, to serve

salt and pepper, to taste

Dressing

1 tbsp extra-virgin olive oil

1 garlic clove, minced

½ tsp honey

pinch cumin, ground

pinch cinnamon, ground

2 tbsp orange juice

Combine the quinoa with 1 cup of water, then bring to the boil and reduce heat to a simmer. Cook for approximately 15 minutes or until the water is absorbed. Let the quinoa sit for 5 minutes and then fluff with a fork.

To make the dressing, in a small bowl whisk together the extra-virgin olive oil, garlic, honey, cumin, cinnamon and orange juice, then set aside.

In a large bowl, toss together the cooked quinoa, segmented orange, beetroot, coriander and almonds. Pour over the dressing, combine well and top with the crumbled cheese. Season to taste.

—

Earthy freekeh also works really well in this recipe. Freekeh is a nutrient-dense grain containing zinc, iron, copper, calcium and magnesium.

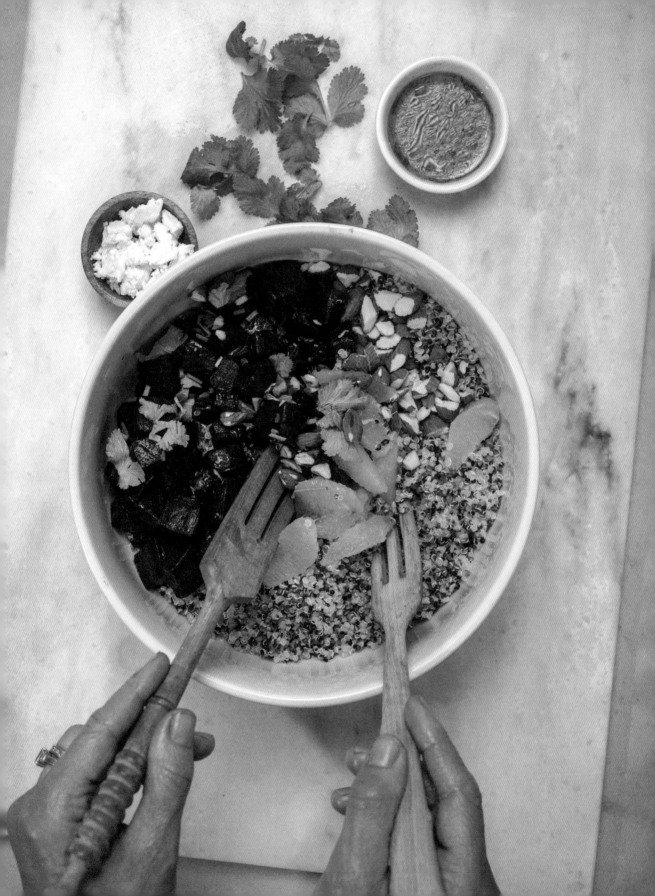

DF, GF, V, VG • **Vitamin C**

Pickled Asian Cabbage Salad

Serves 4 (as a side)
Prep: 15 minutes
Cook: n/a

1½ cups pickled red cabbage

1 carrot, peeled and julienned

1 tbsp fresh ginger, julienned

2 tbsp coriander, chopped

1 tbsp white sesame seeds
  + extra to serve

1 tbsp shallots, finely chopped

¼ cup dry roasted cashews,
  chopped + extra to serve

2 tbsp sesame oil

Combine all of the ingredients in a small bowl and mix well. Sprinkle with the extra sesame seeds and cashews.

—

1 tbsp fresh turmeric grated also works well in this recipe for added anti-inflammatory properties.

DF, GF, V, VG • **Vitamin C**

Pickled Cabbage

Serves 20 (as a condiment)
Prep: 30 minutes
  (+ 1 week pickling time)
Cook: n/a

300 mL apple cider vinegar

½ tbsp salt

300 mL water

1 head small red cabbage,
  shaved finely with a mandolin

1 tsp peppercorns

Place the vinegar, salt and water into a saucepan and bring to the boil.

Place the cabbage and peppercorns in a sterilised jar. Pour in the vinegar brine and place a lid on the jar. Place in a dark cupboard for 1 week. Once opened, stored in the fridge.

—

If preferred, add 1–2 cups cooked quinoa to the salad for added fibre and complex carbohydrates.

DF, GF, V, VG • **Healthy fats**

Vegan Hemp Pesto Sauce

Serves 4
Prep: 5 minutes
Cook: n/a

1 large ripe avocado, seed and skin removed, chopped

½ cup fresh basil leaves

¼ cup unsalted raw macadamia nuts, chopped

1 tbsp hemp seeds

2 tbsp fresh lemon juice

1 tsp lemon zest

2 garlic cloves, crushed

pinch salt and pepper, to taste

Combine all of the ingredients in a food processor and puree until smooth. Add water to thin if needed. Use immediately or store in an airtight container in the fridge for 1 day or freeze.

—

Hemp seed oil can be used in place of hemp seeds if preferred.

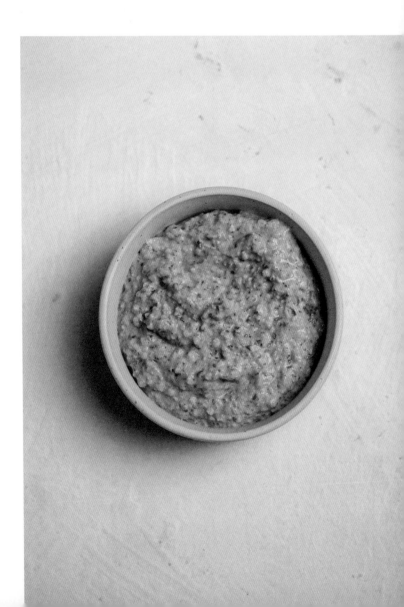

DF, GF, V, VG • **Beta-carotene**

Smoked Paprika Sweet Potato Chips

Serves 4
Prep: 5 minutes
Cook: 20 minutes

2 large sweet potatoes,
   scrubbed and cut into
   1–2 cm batons

1–2 tbsp extra-virgin olive oil

½–1 tsp sea salt

½–1 tsp smoked paprika,
   ground

Preheat the oven to 180°C. Line a baking tray with baking paper.

In a large bowl, combine the sweet potato, extra-virgin olive oil, salt and smoked paprika, then toss well.

Place the sweet potato on the tray in a single layer and bake for 15–20 minutes until tender and golden.

—

Sprinkle with hemp seeds before roasting as an easy way to boost omega-3 intake. You could make crudités in place of sweet potato chips, using carrot, capsicum, endive or cucumber. You could also try cutting pita bread into triangles and baking until crispy.

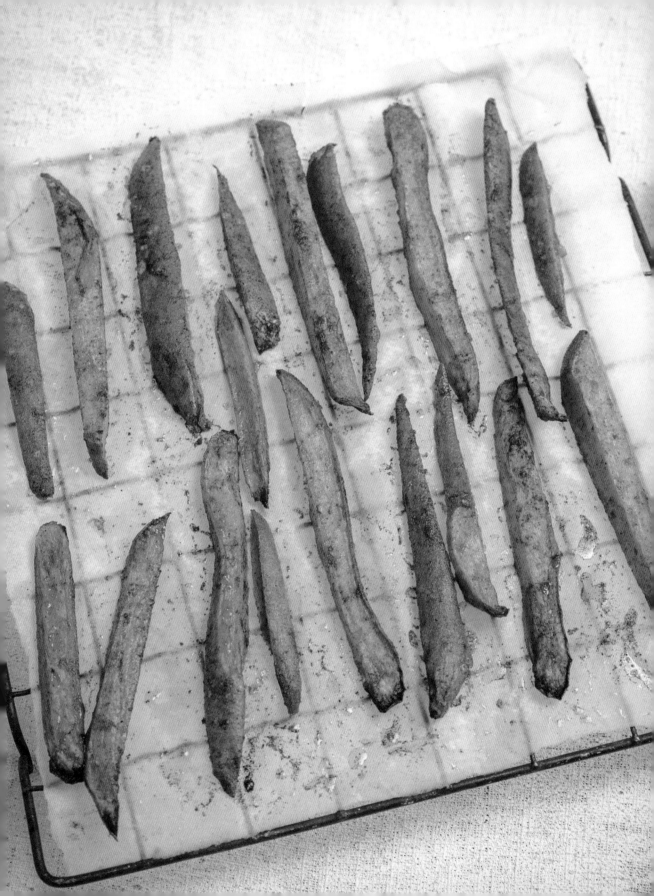

DF, GF, V, VG • Zinc

Zucchini & Chickpea Hummus

Serves 4–6
Prep: 20 minutes
Cook: n/a

1 cup yellow and green zucchini,
  roughly chopped

1 cup chickpeas, cooked

1 cup sunflower seeds, toasted

3 tbsp lemon juice

1 tbsp lemon zest

1 garlic clove

½ cup extra-virgin olive oil

1 tbsp cumin, ground

1 tbsp coriander seeds, ground

1 tbsp good-quality salt

2 cups vegetables, cut into
  sticks, to serve

multigrain crackers (gluten-free
  if required), to serve

Place all of the ingredients apart from the vegetable sticks and crackers in a food processor and blend until smooth.

Serve in a bowl on a platter with the vegetable sticks and crackers.

—

For energy and mood support, try adding 1–2 tsp maca powder before blending.

DF, GF, V • **Antioxidants**

Stir-Fry Sauce

*Makes enough for 400–500 g
 protein
Serves 4–6
Prep: 15 minutes
Cook: n/a*

1 tbsp sesame oil

1 large green chilli, seeds
  removed, thinly sliced

2 garlic cloves, crushed

1 tbsp ginger, grated

2 tbsp miso paste, gluten-free
  + ¼ cup boiling water

2 tbsp tamari soy sauce,
  gluten-free

1 tbsp honey, adjusted to taste

¼ cup mixed herbs (e.g.
  coriander, mint etc)

1 tbsp hemp seeds

virgin coconut oil, melted/
  extra-virgin olive oil, to thin
  if needed

Place all of the ingredients into a small bowl or jar, then mix
until smooth.

Use straight away or store in a jar in the fridge for up to 1 week.

—

*Hemp seeds can be replaced with crushed nuts if preferred –
cashews work well! Miso paste is available from the Asian section
of major supermarkets, Asian grocery stores or health food stores.*

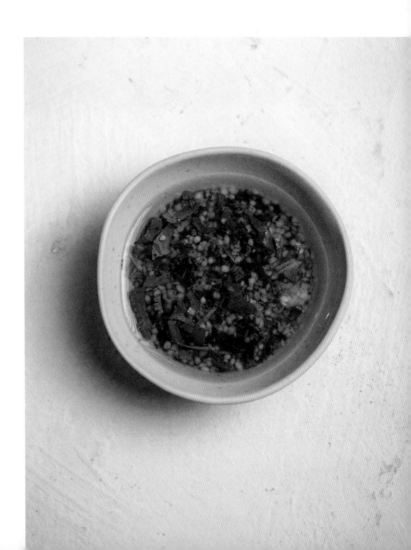

DF, V, VG • Fibre

Zucchini & Asparagus Hemp Seed Crusted Chips – Egg-Free

Serves 4
Prep: 15 minutes
Cook: 15 minutes

½ cup wholemeal breadcrumbs

¼ cup hemp seeds

¼ tsp paprika, ground

1 garlic clove, finely crushed

2 tbsp chia seeds

2 tbsp milk of your choice

3 large zucchini, cut into thick batons

1 bunch asparagus, cut into thick batons

virgin coconut oil/extra-virgin olive, for cooking

sea salt and pepper

In a mixing bowl, add the breadcrumbs, hemp seeds, paprika and garlic.

In a second shallow bowl, mix together the chia seeds and milk.

Dip each piece of zucchini and asparagus into the chia mixture and then into the breadcrumb mix.

Heat the oil in a frying pan over a high heat, then add the zucchini and asparagus in batches and cook for 2 minutes on each side, or until golden. Remove from the pan and place on paper towel.

Sprinkle with the salt and pepper and serve immediately.

—

These chips work really well with Tofu Avocado Mayo (p. 251). These chips are a nice change for kids who love potato chips.

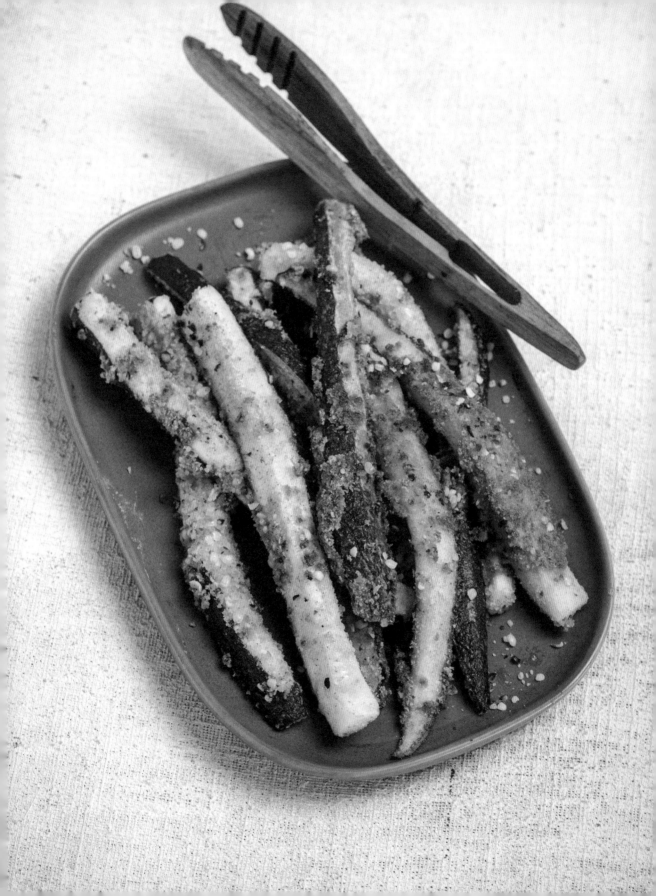

DF, GF, V, VG • **Vitamin C**

Turmeric Cauliflower

Serves 4
Prep: 5 minutes
Cook: 5–6 minutes

1–2 tsp virgin coconut oil

1–2 garlic cloves, crushed

¼ tsp turmeric, ground/
   freshly grated

sea salt and pepper, to taste

2 cups cauliflower, cut into
   florets

½ tbsp lime juice

Heat the coconut oil in a small pan over a medium heat. Add in the garlic and cook for 1 minute. Add the turmeric, salt, pepper and cauliflower and stir until the cauliflower is fully coated with turmeric. Cover the pan with a lid and let cook for 2 minutes. Add the lime juice and stir to coat. Remove from heat and set aside.

—

This recipe also works well with broccoli as an alternative!

DF, GF, V • **Vitamin C**

Roasted Tomato & Vegetable Pasta Sauce

Prep: 15 minutes
Cook: 40 minutes

500 g cherry tomatoes

250 g pumpkin, seeds removed, diced

1 red capsicum, seeds removed, sliced

1 red onion, skin removed, diced

½ tsp chilli flakes, optional

2 tsp paprika, ground

4 garlic cloves, halved

4 tbsp extra-virgin olive oil

1 tsp raw honey, adjusted to taste, optional

1 bunch basil/herbs of your choice, chopped

sea salt and pepper, to taste

Preheat the oven to 180°C. Add the vegetables, spices and garlic to a large roasting tray, then drizzle with the extra-virgin olive oil. Roast for 30–40 minutes until well roasted, when the skin has split and it looks charred.

Remove from the oven and let cool slightly.

Add to a blender with the raw honey and basil, blend until smooth, then season to taste.

Use immediately or store in a glass container in the fridge for up to 5 days, or in the freezer for 3 months.

—

If your kids are sensitive to chilli, this can be left out. This recipe is great for fussy eaters.

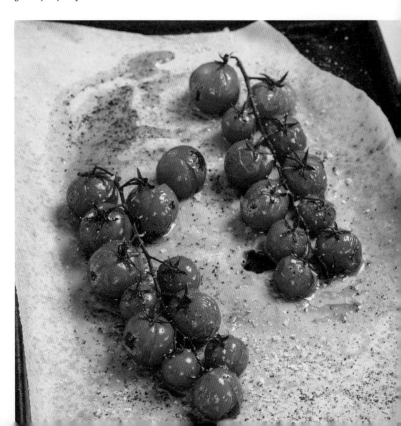

Sweets

V • Protein

Banana Chocolate Muffins with Maple Cream Cheese Frosting

Serves 8–10
Prep: 30 minutes
Cook: 30 minutes

Muffins

½ cup plant-based protein powder

1 tbsp cacao powder

1¼ cups plain wholemeal/ spelt flour

2 tsp baking powder

½ cup almond meal

pinch salt

2 large ripe bananas, mashed

1½ cups almond/cow's milk

2 eggs, lightly beaten

2 tbsp maple syrup

Frosting

250 g cream cheese, softened to room temperature

½ tsp vanilla essence

1 tbsp maple syrup

1–2 tsp milk of your choice

Toppings

banana chips

shaved dark chocolate

Preheat the oven to 160°C and line a muffin tin with patty pans.

In a large bowl, combine the plant-based protein powder, cacao, flour, baking powder, almond meal and salt.

In a small bowl, whisk together the bananas, milk, egg and maple syrup.

Fold the wet mixture into the dry mixture and stir until well combined. Spoon the mixture evenly into the prepared patty pans.

Place the muffin tin in the oven and cook for 20–30 minutes or until a skewer is inserted in the centre and comes out clean. Stand for 5 minutes and transfer to a wire rack to cool.

To make the frosting, beat the cream cheese, vanilla and maple syrup together using an electric mixer until smooth, adding milk slowly until the desired consistency is reached. Adjust sweetness to suit.

Once the muffins are cool, ice with the cream cheese frosting and finish with a banana chip and some shaved dark chocolate.

—

For a dairy-free frosting option, use the cashew icing from Carrot Mini Muffins with Cashew Icing (p. 280).

DF, GF, V, VG • Carbohydrates

Acai Sea Salt Chocolate Crackles

Makes 12
Prep: 10 minutes (+ 30 minutes
  setting time)
Cook: 10 minutes

Chocolate Crackles

300 g virgin coconut oil, melted

2–3 tbsp maple syrup/raw
  honey

4–5 tbsp cacao/cocoa powder

1 tbsp acai powder, optional

½–1 tsp sea salt

2 tbsp plant-based protein
  powder, optional

4 cups puffed rice/quinoa

To Serve

acai/cacao powder, for dusting

mixed fresh berries

Line a muffin tin with patty pans.

In a medium saucepan, add the virgin coconut oil, maple syrup or honey, cocoa or cacao powder, acai powder, sea salt and protein powder. Stir over a low heat until melted and the mixture is well combined.

Add the puffed rice or quinoa to a large mixing bowl. Pour the chocolate mixture into the bowl and combine until all of the puffed rice or quinoa is well covered.

Spoon the mixture into the lined patty pans.

Place in the fridge or freezer until set, for a minimum 30 minutes in the fridge.

To serve, dust with the extra cacao or acai powder and top with the berries.

—

Drizzle these crackles with nut butter for added healthy fats that help to curb sugar cravings. Acai powder can be purchased in the health section of major supermarkets, at health food stores or chemists. This recipe is great for kids' birthday parties.

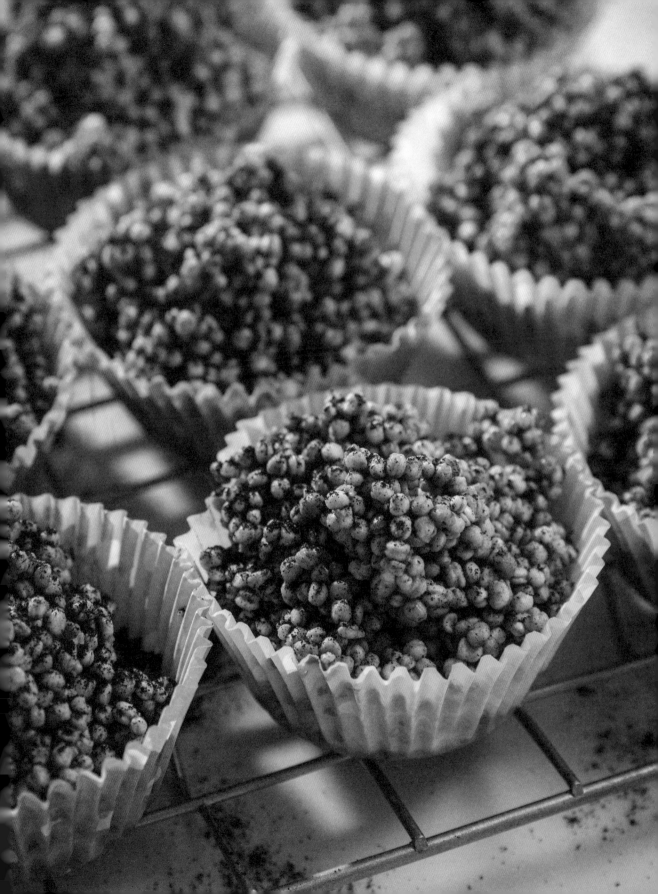

DF, GF, V • **Antioxidants**

Acai Berry & Chocolate Soufflé Sweet Omelette

Serves 1
Prep: 30 minutes
Cook: 10–15 minutes

Soufflé Omelette

2 eggs, yolks and whites
    separated

¼–½ tbsp cacao powder +
    extra to serve

1–2 tsp acai powder + extra
    to serve

1 tbsp almond/coconut milk

honey, optional

½ tbsp virgin coconut oil,
    for cooking

To Serve

natural/coconut yoghurt

fresh berries

mint leaves

Preheat the oven to 180°C.

In a bowl, whisk together the egg yolks, cacao powder, acai powder, milk and optional honey.

In a separate bowl, beat the egg whites until stiff peaks form.

Gently fold the egg whites into the cacao mixture and combine.

Heat the virgin coconut oil in a small ovenproof frying pan over a medium heat, pour the mixture into the pan and cook for a few minutes until it begins to set. Place under a hot grill in the oven for 5 minutes to finish cooking.

Top the soufflé omelette with the yoghurt, fresh berries, mint leaves and an extra sprinkle of the cacao powder and acai powder.

—

For added fibre and healthy fats, stir 1 tbsp LSA into the yoghurt before serving alongside the omelette! Acai powder can be purchased in the health section of major supermarkets, at health food stores or chemists.

GF, V • **B vitamins**

Buckwheat & Maca Crepes with Honey Whipped Ricotta & Roasted Berries

Serves 4
Prep: 30 minutes
  (+ 30 minutes standing time)
Cook: 40 minutes

Buckwheat Crepes

1 cup buckwheat flour, sifted

2 tsp organic maca powder

1 cup cow's/almond/coconut milk

1 tbsp honey

1 egg, lightly beaten

pinch salt

1 tbsp coconut oil, melted + extra for cooking

Roasted Berries

2 cups mixed berries

1 tbsp honey

Honey Whipped Ricotta

200 g ricotta cheese

1–2 tbsp honey

1 tbsp lemon juice

1–2 tsp lemon zest

For the crepes, whisk all of the ingredients (except the coconut oil) in a large bowl until a batter forms. Let stand at room temperature for 30 minutes.

To make the roasted berries, preheat the oven to 180°C. Combine all of the ingredients in an ovenproof dish and bake for 15–20 minutes until the berries start to break down. Remove from the oven, then set aside.

For the whipped ricotta, combine the ricotta, honey and lemon juice in a food processor, blend until smooth, taste for sweetness. Stir through the lemon zest. Set aside in the fridge.

To cook the crepes, heat the coconut oil in a non-stick pan. Pour in enough batter to almost cover the base of the pan and swirl the pan so that the batter is even. When bubbles appear on the surface, flip the crepe and cook on the other side. Repeat with remaining mixture.

To serve, spread the ricotta mix over 1 side of the crepe. Top with the berries and roll up to enclose the filling. Repeat with the remaining crepes.

—

For a dairy-free alternative, swap ricotta cheese for coconut yoghurt. Maca powder can be purchased in the health section of major supermarkets, at health food stores or chemists.

GF, V • Vitamin E

Extra-Virgin Olive Oil Orange Cake

Serves 8–12
Prep: 10–15 minutes
Cook: 40 minutes

Orange Cake

250 g honey

3 eggs

1 tsp sea salt

250 mL extra-virgin olive oil

250 mL cow's milk

150 mL fresh orange juice

1 tbsp orange zest

500 g almond flour

1 tbsp baking powder

Vanilla Yoghurt

200 mL coconut yoghurt

1 vanilla bean/1 tsp vanilla
   bean paste

Orange Decoration

1 orange, cut into thin slices

1 tbsp extra-virgin olive oil

½ tsp cinnamon, ground

1 tbsp maple syrup/honey

Preheat the oven to 180°C. Line a circular cake tin with baking paper.

In a large bowl, mix together the honey, eggs and sea salt.

In a second bowl, combine the extra-virgin olive oil, milk, orange juice and zest and gently mix.

Combine all the wet ingredients in the large bowl, then fold through the flour and baking powder. Pour into the cake tin.

Cook for 20–25 minutes or until golden brown.

Mix together the yoghurt and vanilla bean, then set aside.

For the orange decoration, mix ingredients together in a bowl, place in a baking dish and bake for 15 minutes at 180°C or until golden brown.

Once the cake is cooked, decorate with baked orange slices and serve with a dollop of vanilla yoghurt on top.

—

For a dairy-free version, use oat or almond milk in place of cow's milk.

V • Magnesium

Cacao Beet Brownies

Serves 10
Prep: 20 minutes
Cook: 30 minutes

2 large beetroots, peeled, diced and cooked

3 eggs, lightly beaten

½ cup coconut sugar

¼ cup wholemeal plain flour

¼ tsp baking powder

⅓ cup cacao powder

⅓ cup hazelnut/almond meal

1 tbsp beetroot powder

100 g dark chocolate, roughly chopped

1 tbsp virgin coconut oil, melted

Preheat the oven to 160°C. Lightly grease and line a 20 × 20 cm baking tray with baking paper.

Add the beetroot to a food processor or blender and blend until smooth, then set aside.

In a large bowl, using electric beaters, beat the eggs and sugar until light and fluffy. Sift the flour, baking powder and cacao powder over the mixture, then fold in well. Add the hazelnut or almond meal, beetroot powder, dark chocolate and coconut oil, and combine well.

Pour into the prepared baking tray and cook for 20–30 minutes until slightly firm to touch, or a skewer comes out clean.

—

For a bit of crunch, add ⅓ cup chopped walnuts or hazelnuts to the mix. Beetroot powder can be purchased in the health section of major supermarkets, at health food stores or chemists.

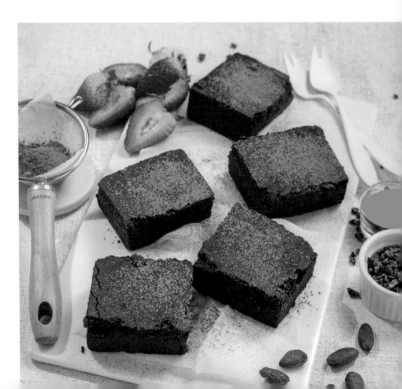

DF, V • **Healthy fats**

Carrot Mini Muffins with Cashew Icing

Makes 10–12 mini muffins
Prep: 30 minutes (+ 4–6 hours or
  overnight soaking cashews)
Cook: 20–25 minutes

Mini Muffins

3 eggs

½ cup honey/maple syrup

2 carrots, grated

100 g almond meal

¼ cup wholemeal plain flour

½ cup wholemeal self-raising
  flour

¼ cup milk of your choice

Cashew Butter Icing

150 g raw cashews, pre-soaked
  for 4–6 hours/overnight

½–1 tbsp honey/maple syrup,
  adjusted to taste

2 tbsp milk of your choice/
  melted coconut oil + extra if
  needed

½ tbsp orange zest

Preheat the oven to 180°C and grease mini muffin tins.

In a bowl, place the eggs and honey, then beat with an electric mixer until light and creamy.

Stir through the carrots, almond meal, flours and milk. Mix well and spoon into the muffin tins.

Bake for 20–25 minutes, or until cooked through. Let cool.

To make the icing, drain the cashews and place in a blender alongside the honey or maple syrup, milk and orange zest. Blend until smooth and desired consistency is reached, adding additional milk as needed.

Spread a dollop of icing on each mini muffin.

—

Try sneaking in some grated zucchini for added fibre! Get kids involved with icing the muffins.

DF, V, VG • **Prebiotics**

Chai Spiced Apple Crumble with Honey Cinnamon Yoghurt

Serves 6–8
Prep: 20 minutes
Cook: 45 minutes

Crumble

2 cups oats

1 cup almond meal

⅓ cup shredded coconut

½ cup dates, seeds removed, finely chopped

¼ tsp each – cardamom, all spice, nutmeg and cloves, ground

½ tsp each – cinnamon and ginger, ground

2 tbsp coconut oil, melted

Apple Mixture

6 green apples, peeled and cut into 2 cm cubes

½ tbsp honey/maple syrup

1 cup water

Honey Cinnamon Yoghurt

2 cups natural Greek yoghurt/ coconut yoghurt

1–2 tbsp honey/maple syrup

pinch cinnamon, ground

Preheat the oven to 180°C.

In a bowl, combine the oats, almond meal, coconut, dates and spices, and mix well. Add melted coconut oil and rub the mixture together using your fingertips until a crumb forms.

Tip the crumble mixture onto a lined baking tray and spread out evenly. Cook for 15 minutes until lightly golden, then remove from the oven and set side.

To make the apple mixture, place the apple, honey or maple syrup and water into a saucepan. Bring to the boil and simmer for 10 minutes until the apples are tender and the water has evaporated. Set aside.

Whisk together the yoghurt, honey and cinnamon. Adjust sweetness to suit, then set aside.

In a medium baking dish, layer the apple and chia crumble mix and bake in the oven for 10 minutes, or until golden brown and bubbling.

Serve with the honey cinnamon yoghurt.

—

Apples are a good source of polyphenols – a class of chemical compounds found within plants, which exert antioxidant activities in the body, helping to neutralise free radicals from oxidative stress and inflammation.

V • **Carbohydrates**

Chocolate & Coconut-Dipped Frozen Fruit

Serves 10
Prep: 40 minutes (+ 30 minutes
  freezing time)
Cook: 20 minutes

Toppings

crushed nuts

hemp seeds

coconut

sprinkles

Chocolate Sauce

200 g chocolate, chopped

2 tbsp coconut cream

1 tsp pure vanilla extract

Skewers

diced fruit of your choice
  (e.g. strawberries, pineapple,
  banana etc), pre-frozen with
  sticks/skewers

Line 1–2 baking sheets with baking paper.

Pour toppings of your choice onto plates.

Add the chocolate to a heatproof bowl placed over a pot of boiling water. Continually stir until the chocolate has melted. Stir in the coconut cream and vanilla extract. Turn the heat to low.

Take the fruit from the freezer and start dipping the fruit into the chocolate, twirling to make sure the fruit is well covered. Roll in toppings and place on the baking sheet. Repeat.

Place back in the freezer for 15–30 minutes until the chocolate has set.

—

This recipe also works well with dried fruit and is a great way to get kids involved and engaged with cooking.

DF, GF, V, VG • **Antioxidants**

Mango, Pawpaw & Pear Fruit Salad with Banana Sauce & Roasted Coconut

Serves 2–4
Prep: 15 minutes
Cook: 5–10 minutes

Fruit Salad

100 g coconut slivers

½ cup pawpaws, diced

½ cup pears, diced

½ cup mangoes, diced

1 orange, segmented

Banana Sauce

2 ripe bananas

juice of ½ lemon

juice of ½ lime

¼ cup mint

Preheat the oven to 180°C. Place the coconut slivers on a baking tray and bake for 5 minutes, or until golden brown.

To make the sauce, place the banana, lemon juice, lime juice and mint in a food processor and process until smooth.

In a bowl, gently mix the pawpaw, pear, mango and orange.

Place the fruit mixture into individual bowls and pour over the banana dressing. Sprinkle with the coconut slivers to finish and serve in decorative glasses.

—

For added decadence, grate dark chocolate over the fruit salad before serving.

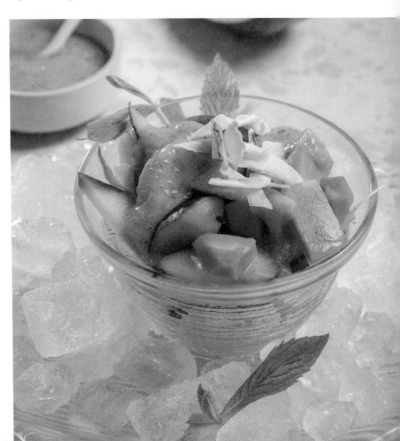

DF, GF, V • **Healthy fats**

Gluten-Free Strawberry & Hazelnut Muffins

Serves 6
Prep: 30 minutes
Cook: 40 minutes

1 cup fresh/frozen strawberries, stems removed, diced + extra slices for topping

1 tbsp honey

½ cup hazelnut/almond meal

1 cup coconut flour/buckwheat flour

½ tsp cinnamon, ground

1½ tsp baking powder

1 egg, lightly beaten

1 cup coconut/almond/cow's milk

1 tsp vanilla essence

½ cup extra-virgin olive oil/ coconut oil + extra to thin if needed

dollop of coconut/Greek yoghurt, to serve, optional

Preheat the oven to 180°C and grease or individually line muffin tins.

In a small saucepan, add the strawberries and honey and stew for 5 minutes, or until the strawberries have softened. Mash slightly then remove from the heat and leave to cool.

In a large mixing bowl, combine the hazelnut or almond meal, flour, cinnamon and baking powder. In a small bowl, whisk together the egg, milk, vanilla essence and oil. Add the wet mixture to the dry mixture and combine well before folding in the strawberry mixture.

Spoon the batter into the greased muffin tins and top each with a slice of fresh strawberry.

Cook for 25–30 minutes for large muffins or 10 minutes for mini muffins, or until a skewer is inserted and comes out clean.

Remove from the trays once cool and store in an airtight container. If freezing, drizzle each muffin with a small amount of oil first to maintain moisture when defrosting.

The muffins are best served warm with a dollop of yoghurt and topped with the extra strawberry slices.

—

For a nut-free option, swap hazelnut or almond meal for sunflower, flax meal or pepita meal.

DF, GF, V, VG • **Magnesium**

Homemade Chocolate Nut Coconut Bars

Serves 20
*Prep: 10 minutes (+ 1 hour
    freezing time)*
Cook: n/a

70 g cocoa/cacao powder

60 g chocolate plant-based
    protein powder

1 cup extra-virgin coconut oil,
    melted

75 g almond butter

100 g almond meal

100 g coconut flour

2 scoops stevia powder/
    2–4 tbsp raw honey, optional

1 pinch chilli powder, optional

50 g shredded coconut + extra
    for topping

dash vanilla essence

In a large mixing bowl, combine all of the ingredients.

Line a square or rectangle baking dish at least 2 cm high with baking paper. Pour the mixture into the baking dish and sprinkle with the extra coconut over the top. Place in the freezer for approximately 60 minutes or until set.

Remove from the freezer and cut into bite-sized pieces.

—

If suffering hot flashes, omit chilli powder and replace with turmeric and cinnamon.

DF, GF, V • **Protein**

Lemon Poppy Seed Protein Pancakes

Serves 1
Prep: 15 minutes
Cook: 10 minutes

Pancakes

2 tbsp vanilla plant-based
  protein powder

1 pinch baking powder

1 tbsp shredded coconut,
  toasted

1 pinch salt

1 large/2 small eggs, beaten

2 tbsp water, if needed

1–2 tbsp fresh lemon juice

2 tsp lemon zest

1 tsp poppy seeds

2 tsp extra-virgin olive oil

To Serve

1½ tbsp coconut yoghurt

blueberries

In a mixing bowl, combine the protein powder, baking powder, coconut and salt, then mix well. In a second bowl, mix together the eggs, water, lemon juice and zest. Combine the wet mixture with the dry mixture and stir through the poppy seeds.

Heat the extra-virgin olive oil in a frying pan over a medium heat. Add spoonfuls of pancake batter to the pan and cook for a few minutes or until bubbles appear. Flip and cook for a further 2 minutes. Repeat with the remaining mixture.

Pile the pancakes onto a plate and top with the yoghurt and blueberries.

—

As a chocolate craving buster, use chocolate protein powder and/ or add a sprinkle of cacao nibs into the pancake batter.

DF, GF, V, VG • **Protein**

Lemon Hemp Bliss Balls

Makes 8–10 balls
Prep: 30 minutes
Cook: n/a

½ cup hemp seeds + extra
  for coating

1 cup almond meal

2 cups shredded coconut

juice of ½ lemon

zest of 1 lemon/lime/orange

1 tsp vanilla bean paste

½ cup dates, seeds removed

½ tsp sea salt

water, to thin if needed

Place all of the ingredients into a food processor and mix until well combined.

Place the extra hemp seeds onto a plate. Remove the blades from the processor and roll a heaped tablespoon of the mixture into balls using your hands. Toss the balls in the hemp seeds until well covered. Place the balls into an airtight container and refrigerate.

—

These bliss balls are high in healthy fats, so a great option mid-afternoon to quash sugar cravings.

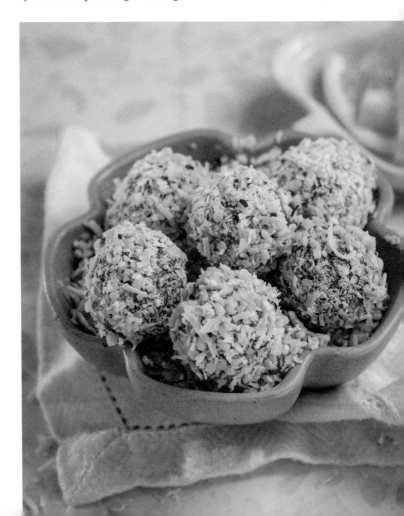

V • **Antioxidants**

Mini Dark Chocolate & Beetroot Lava Pudding

Serves 8
Prep: 15 minutes
Cook: 15 minutes

Lava Pudding

180 g dark chocolate, chopped

250 g virgin coconut oil

4 eggs

½ cup honey/maple syrup

½ tbsp beetroot powder

¼ cup spelt plain flour, sifted

Topping

spoonful coconut yoghurt

fresh berries

Combine the dark chocolate and virgin coconut oil in a small saucepan over a low heat, stirring until melted. Set aside to cool.

Preheat the oven to 180°C. Grease 8 × 175 mL ceramic ovenproof dishes and sprinkle with a little bit of flour to prevent the puddings from sticking.

Using an electric mixer, beat the eggs and honey or maple syrup for 10 minutes, or until thick and creamy. Fold in the chocolate mixture, beetroot powder and spelt flour. Spoon the mixture into prepared dishes.

Place the dishes on a baking tray. Bake for 10 minutes, or until just set.

Stand the dishes for 30 seconds. Turn onto plates and top with the coconut yoghurt and berries.

—

Acai powder can be used in place of beetroot powder if preferred. Both acai and beetroot powder can be purchased in the health section of major supermarkets, at health food stores or chemists.

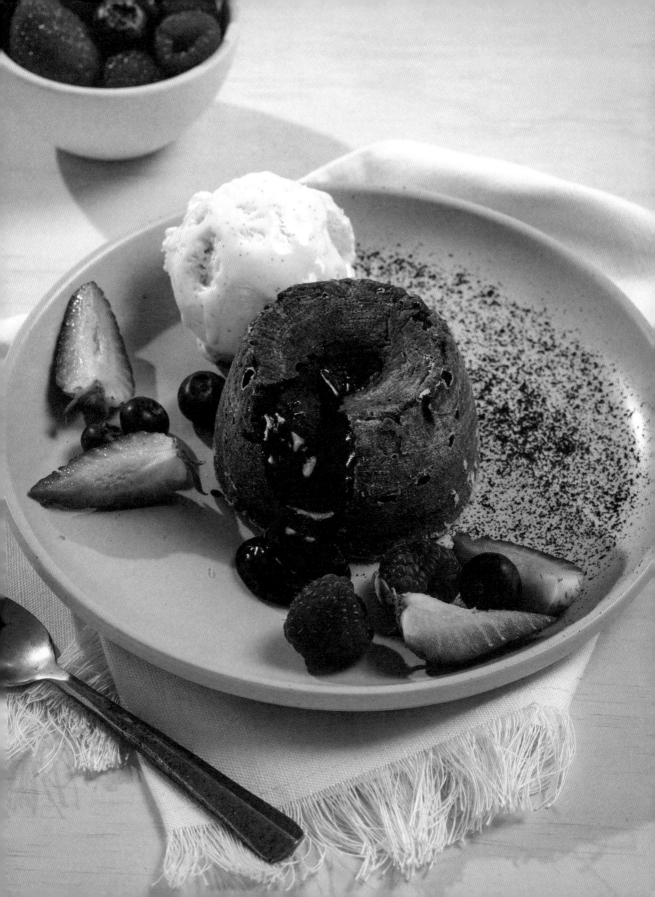

DF, GF, V • **Fibre**

Pear, Banana & Blueberry Muffins

Makes 8–12 muffins
Prep: 20 minutes
Cook: 20–30 minutes

4 eggs

¼ cup extra-virgin olive oil

2–3 small ripe bananas

1–2 small pears, core removed

½ cup blueberries

½ tsp vanilla extract

½ cup pepitas/pumpkin seeds,
  optional

½ tsp cinnamon, ground

½ cup tapioca flour

1¼ cup buckwheat flour

1 tsp baking powder

Preheat the oven to 180°C.

In a bowl, mix the wet ingredients together. In a second bowl, mix the dry ingredients together. Gently pour the 2 together – don't use a blender, as it will stop it rising.

Line a muffin tin with patty pans and spoon the batter into each muffin hole.

Cook for 20–30 minutes or until golden brown and cooked through.

—

As a morning or afternoon snack, have these muffins with a dandelion root 'coffee'. Dandelion is a potent liver tonic, which helps to regulate and support the body's natural detoxification processes.

DF, GF, V, VG • **Carbohydrates**

Pumpkin & Banana Brown Rice Muffins with Strawberries

Serves up to 12
Prep: 20 minutes
Cook: 20–25 minutes

Muffins

100 g buckwheat flour

150 g brown rice flour

1 tsp baking powder

1 tsp cinnamon, ground

3 ripe bananas, mashed

1 tsp vanilla extract

1 cup pumpkin, steamed and mashed

200 mL cow's/coconut milk

½ cup extra-virgin olive oil/ rice bran oil

Topping

coconut/Greek yoghurt

1 punnet strawberries, finely chopped

Preheat the oven to 180°C. Place patty pans into a 12-pan muffin tin.

Combine all the dry ingredients in a mixing bowl. In a separate bowl, combine the mashed bananas, vanilla extract, mashed pumpkin, milk and oil. Add the dry ingredients to the banana mixture and mix to combine.

Spoon the batter into the patty pans and bake for 20–25 minutes or until a skewer is inserted in the middle of the muffins and comes out clean.

Top the muffins with the yoghurt and fresh strawberries.

—

These muffins make a yummy lunchbox addition or after-school snack. The pumpkin not only adds a touch of sweetness, but also more fibre along with vitamin C and beta-carotene, both of which help to support immunity.

GF, V • **Antioxidants**

Yoghurt Panna Cotta with Acai Nuts & Syrup

Serves 6–8
Prep: 20 minutes
  (+ 4 hours setting time)
Cook: 30 minutes

Panna Cotta

½ cup milk of your choice

½ tbsp vanilla essence

2 tsp agar agar

1 tbsp maple syrup

1½ cups natural Greek yoghurt

Acai Nut Crumb

2 tsp acai powder

4 fresh dates, seeds removed,
  roughly chopped

⅓ cup almond meal

⅓ cup shredded coconut

⅓ cup macadamia nuts,
  chopped

1–2 tbsp maple syrup

Acai Syrup

½ tsp acai powder

3 tbsp honey

3 tbsp water

Place the milk in a small saucepan over a low heat. Add the vanilla essence and agar agar and stir until dissolved. Take off the heat and allow the mixture to cool.

Whisk in the maple syrup and yoghurt. Pour the mixture into individual ½ cup moulds and refrigerate until firm, for approximately 4 hours.

To make the nut crumb, combine the acai powder, dates, almond meal, coconut and macadamia nuts in a food processor and pulse until the nuts are chopped. Slowly add the maple syrup and continue to pulse until the mixture resembles a crumb, then set aside.

Place the acai syrup ingredients in a small saucepan and reduce to a syrup consistency, or until it covers the back of a spoon.

To serve, place a panna cotta in the centre of a plate, sprinkle with the nut crumb around the outside and drizzle with the acai syrup.

—

Acai is a source of antioxidant compounds – especially anthocyanins, which protect the body against free radical damage. Acai powder can be purchased in the health section of major supermarkets, at health food stores or chemists.

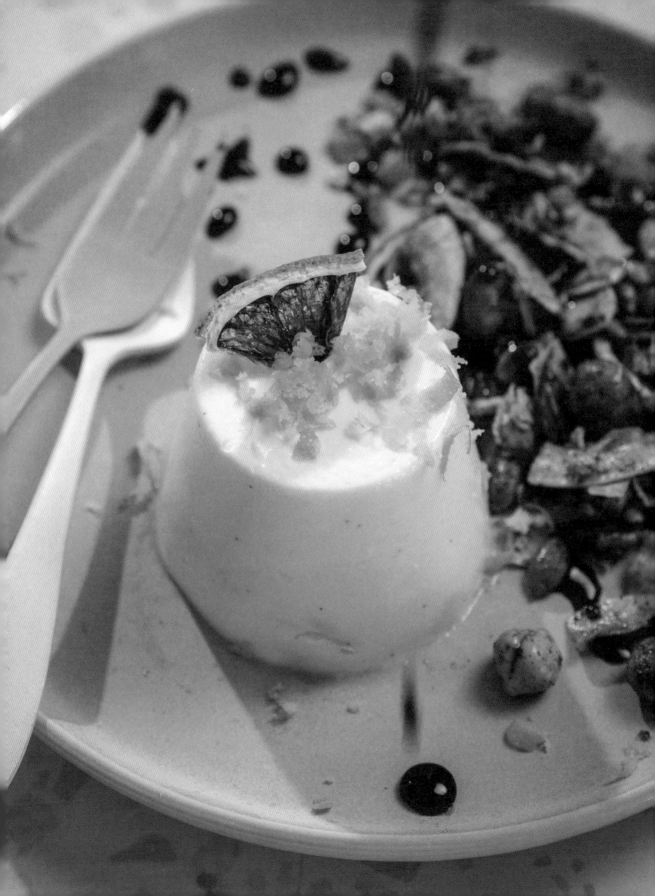

Acknowledgements

Firstly, I want to acknowledge my mum, Judy, for being the ultimate health food guru and sparking my passion for nutritious cooking. I also want to thank my dad, Bing, for encouraging me to go to Le Cordon Bleu in London – I ended up putting on 10 kilos from being a poor student and eating all the leftovers I'd cooked. This compelled me to then work in the south of France to learn about fresh provincial food, the wonder of taste and the positive impact they can have on your health. I have always kept that curiosity with me. Thank you, Trish Robinson, for this life-changing experience of getting to know French food.

A massive thank you to my hubby for always pushing me to be my best, in the kitchen and beyond. And to my little sous-chef, Emily, thanks for your adventurous palate and endless questions – you really make me think.

To all the readers embarking on this health adventure with me, I extend my warmest thanks for your support and enthusiasm. I hope this book may help start you down a very positive journey.

General Index

Recipe Index

Note: Page numbers in bold show items in sample meal plans.

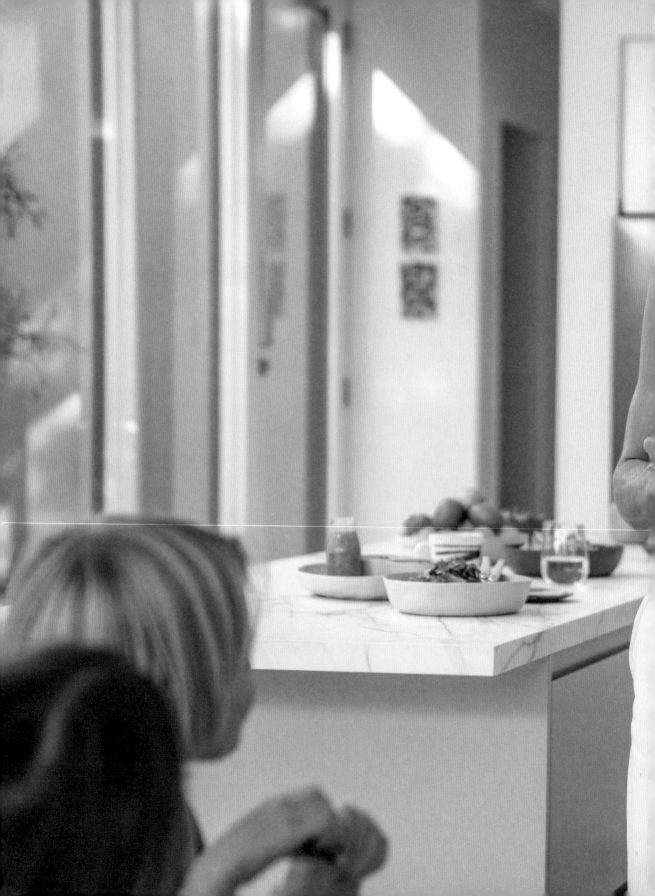

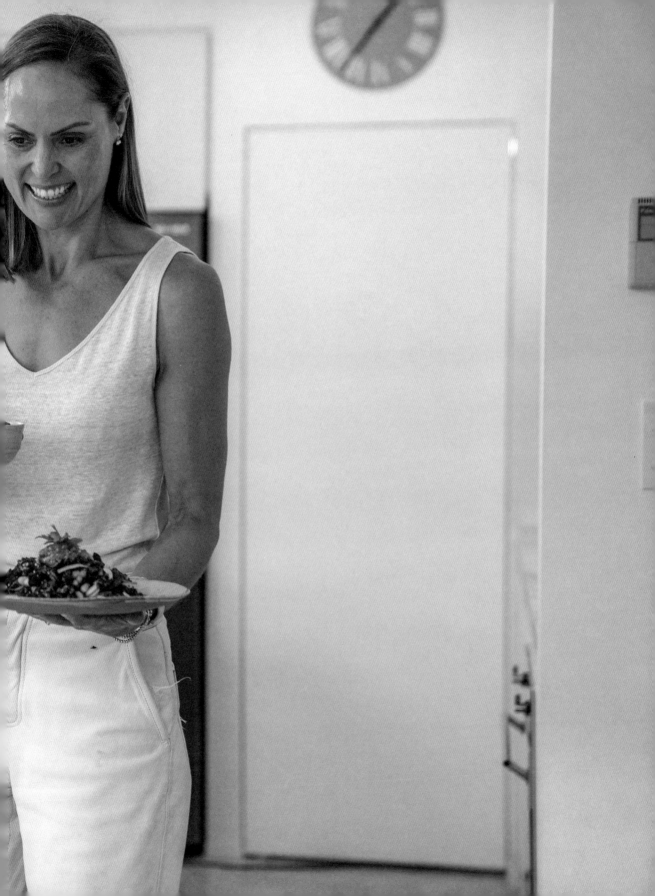

affirm press

First published by Affirm Press in 2024
Bunurong/Boon Wurrung Country
28 Thistlethwaite Street
South Melbourne VIC 3205
affirmpress.com.au

10 9 8 7 6 5 4 3 2 1

The information in this book is general in nature. Please consult your healthcare
practitioner before making any dietary or lifestyle changes, to ensure you choose
the approach that works best for you.

A catalogue record for this
book is available from the
National Library of Australia

ISBN: 9781922992512 (paperback)

Cover design by Andy Warren © Affirm Press
Internal design by Emily Thiang © Affirm Press
Printed in China by C&C Offset Printing Co., Ltd.

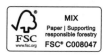